· THE AIDS · CAREGIVER'S HANDBOOK

· THE AIDS ·
CAREGIVER'S
HANDBOOK

EDITED BY TED EIDSON

ST. MARTIN'S PRESS

■ NEW YORK ■

Grateful acknowledgment is made to the following people and organizations for permission to quote from their materials:

BettyClare Moffatt, IBS Press, and National American Library Books for permission to quote from *When Someone You Love Has AIDS: A Book of Hope for Family and Friends*, copyright © 1986, IBS Press; copyright © 1987, New American Library.

Michael Shernoff, Dixie Beckham, Luis Palacios, Vincent Patti, and Chelsea Psychotherapy Associates for permission to reprint in Appendix A "When a Friend Has AIDS," copyright © 1984, Chelsea Psychotherapy Associates.

Kris MacDonald, M.D., editor, for permission to reprint in Appendix A "Evidence of Lack of HTLV-III Transmission Among Families" from the Minnesota Disease Control Newsletter.

Helen Schietinger and Grace Lusby for permission to reprint in Appendix A "Infection Precautions for Those Giving Direct Care to People with AIDS in the Home," revised September 1986.

Michael Helquist and the San Francisco AIDS Foundation for permission to reprint in Appendix B "Getting Your Affairs in Order," copyright © 1983, Michael Helquist and the San Francisco AIDS Foundation.

Design by Judy Stagnitto

Library of Congress Cataloging-in-Publication Data

The AIDS caregiver's handbook / Ted Eidson, editor; introduction by
    BettyClare Moffatt. —Rev. ed.
        p. cm.
    Includes bibliographical references and index.
    ISBN 0-312-08129-4 (pbk.)
    ISBN 0-312-08497-8 (hc)
    1. AIDS (Disease)—Nursing—Handbooks, manuals, etc.
    2. Caregivers—Handbooks, manuals, etc.   I. Eidson, Ted.
    [DNLM: 1. Acquired Immunodeficiency Syndrome—handbooks.
    2. Caregivers—handbooks.   WD 301 A288]
    RC607.A26A34572 1992
    616.97'92—dc20
    DNLM/DLC
    for Library of Congress   92-49770
                                                                    CIP

10 9 8 7 6 5 4 3 2 1

This book is dedicated with love and appreciation for the life of

■ HOWIE DAIRE ■

Founder of the Oak Lawn Counseling Center and, later, of its AIDS Projects. He taught us how to live proudly, to love and care for others, and to work together toward community mental health; and during his death process from various AIDS-related ailments, he showed us that dying can be as exciting and rewarding as living, that it is just another stage of growth.

The writers and editor of this book have donated 25 percent of the royalties from the book to the Harold P. Daire Memorial Fund, P.O. Box 191094, Dallas, Texas 75219.

■ CONTENTS ■

various women's HIV support groups. Discussion of the particular needs of HIV-infected women: psychosocially, medically, and practically.

When a Friend Has AIDS by Dixie Beckham, Luis Palacios, Vincint Patti, and Michael Shernoff, copyright © 1984 by Chelsea Psychotherapy Associates; Evidence of Lack of HTLV-III Transmission Among Families by Kris Macdonald, M.D., in the Minnesota Disease Control Newsletter; Infection Precautions for Those Giving Direct Care to People with AIDS in the Home by Helen Schietinger, M.A., R.N. and Grace Lusby, M.S., R.N.

Getting Your Affairs in Order by Michael Helquist, copyright © 1983 by The San Francisco AIDS Foundation; Rights of People with AIDS; Medical Consent Form (Sample); Solemn Statement Regarding Death (Sample).

Generic List of Local and National Groups; National Telephone Hotlines; Other Sources of Information and Referrals.

Reading List; Cassettes; Addresses of Smaller Publishers and Cassette Distributors; Subscriptions; Workshops.

The editor wishes especially to thank: BettyClare Moffatt for her continued encouragement; Joe Fleming for allowing himself to be a soundingboard and for the storyline in the grief section, Chapter 12; the Dallas County Health Department's AIDS Prevention Project for continuing information and support; and Gene Klump for his unfailing belief in this project and me.

▪ FOREWORD ▪

The Oak Lawn Counseling Center has been a focal point in the Dallas area for the past five years for educational and training materials relating to Acquired Immune Deficiency Syndrome. As the disease spreads, the Center receives more calls from areas newly afflicted with AIDS or individuals who, though outside our area, know of no other place to contact. As others have shared freely with us, we share willingly with others.

But as the case load in Dallas increases, we have less available time to share; indeed we often are not able to meet our local needs with the manpower or expediency we would want. This book, therefore, is designed to impart as much training information as we can so that any individual, health-care professional, or group will know what to do with their own friends or loved ones who are diagnosed with AIDS or ARC (AIDS-Related Complex).

The AIDS Caregiver's Handbook is a compilation of the material that is presented in a two-and-a-half-day training seminar to those who decide to become volunteer caregivers or those who have been tossed into the maelstrom by virtue of their personal relationship with the AIDS or ARC patient. All of the information is directed toward an individual caregiver; thus the information is equally valid for a mother or lover who must take care of an afflicted person as for the members of a hospital staff who have individual responsibilities on an AIDS ward.

The AIDS Caregiver's Handbook is designed to accomplish two ends: to tell you what you must know right now to assist a person with AIDS or ARC; and to tell you where to find more information when you have the time and desire. In this sense, the *Handbook* is more akin to a first aid manual, easily read and easily referenced, than to a medical textbook.

Unless the spread of the Human Immunodeficiency Virus (HIV) can be arrested and everyone presently infected cured in the next couple of years, this book will need to be revised to present up-to-date information. Suggested changes for future editions would be greatly appreciated. Please address them to:

Ted Eidson
Valley AIDS Council
2220 Haine Drive, Ste. 33
Harlingen, TX 78550
(512) 428-9322

■INTRODUCTION■

BETTYCLARE MOFFATT

When I first read the manuscript of *The AIDS Caregiver's Handbook*, I wept. But they were tears of joy. I could see so clearly the individual and collective compassion behind the words on paper. I could see an army of caregivers and PWAs reaching out to help us all; in some ways, to walk through our grief into a process of gratitude for our own changed lives.

For *The AIDS Caregiver's Handbook* is a book of service, of serviceable love. As such, I am honored to share a part of myself in its pages. I did not always feel this way.

If anyone had told me, just four years ago, that I would be working in the field of AIDS Education and AIDS awareness, writing, lecturing, publishing, and counseling, I would have looked at that person as if he had just stepped off of the planet Mars, and asked stupidly, "AIDS? What is AIDS?"

My mind would have leaped, perhaps to aid to starving children in Biafra, or helping the homeless with a hot meal or a place to lay their heads, or aid to dependent children; to "aiding," in other words, those people "out there," far from my safe world as a (then) suburban Texas housewife, mother/grandmother, writer/teacher. I was innocent.

I am innocent no more. In *When Someone You Love Has AIDS: A Book of Hope for Family and Friends*, I wrote in anguish: "You must go through your feelings about AIDS no matter how painful the process, no matter how long it takes. For when someone you love has AIDS, there is no place to run, no place to hide. We survive, and help our loved one. Or we go under."

My son, Michael Welsch, contracted AIDS in the spring of 1984. He died July 14, 1986, in San Francisco, surrounded by his loving family. Michael was one of the lucky ones. He had family, friends, an understanding boss, and good medical and home care. He had a chance to come to terms mentally, physically, emotionally, and spiritually with his life and ultimately, his death.

Many who have AIDS are not so fortunate. Many of the caregivers who have watched friends, lovers, husbands, wives, and children die of this implacable, incomprehensible, ugly disease are both burned-out and worn-out. How can we stop the tide of death that keeps rolling in, as heartless and indifferent and awesome as the sea, rolling over us all in a tide of grief and exhaustion? We are forced daily to examine our beliefs about life, about death, about sexuality, about plague. We face prejudice along with fear and ignorance, and we, like the PWAs, often fight until we drop.

And yet, as Michael wrote so determinedly in *When Someone You Love Has AIDS,* "AIDS is a gift that has awakened me to life." *Life!*

For in the midst of our loved ones' struggles for life in the face of death, it is we who *learn.* We learn how to love in the face of our own failures and fears, within the arena of our anger and our anguish. We learn what is really important to us. And, if we look for it, we find joy. Joy! We find our own private source of strength to share in a public way; we find intense caring; we find luminous moments as flesh gives way to spirit. And we, the caregivers, are healed.

Because of Michael and AIDS, I will never be the same again. Michael and the scores of people like him whom we honor in our lives will be there for me and for you. They are there for the Mothers of AIDS Patients (MAP) groups, which two friends and I co-founded and which is now a national network of emotional support for families and friends of AIDS patients. They are there for the buddy programs such as the ones so movingly detailed in this book. They are there for the Shanti Project and hospice and counseling centers and Caregiver groups everywhere. Their lives are not in vain—never, never, never in vain! For they taught us how to love, and they taught us how to live. They are seeds that fell, and out of their passage, we can move on to help others, so that we who live are enriched and strengthened and honored to be a part of the way home in the midst of this plague on all our houses.

As I go across the country speaking to groups everywhere who are soldiers in this war against AIDS, I see Michael's face shining out from each one. And I feel his strength, his peace, his courage infusing me.

One instance stands out so clearly. It was a buddy-training workshop at Oak Lawn Counseling Center in Dallas, Texas. I had gone from California, where I now live, back to Texas for the occasion. I can still feel the sense of panic that swept over me as I looked at the assembled concerned and caring individuals before me. Michael had died three months before. What in the world was I doing here with a videotape microphone strapped to my sweating waist? What could I possibly say or do that would make any difference? A prepared speech was only words on paper. Words for the survivors, the weary warriors in the battle against AIDS. What could anyone do or say to heal the pain? What could anyone do or say to make it all better?

Michael spoke to me: "Tell the truth, Mama, just tell the truth."

And so I shared with the congregation of caregivers my deepest truths about my own journey through the life and death of my son. And I have continued to tell the truth to anyone and everyone who will listen. It's more about life than it is about death; more about learning to love than anything else.

If it seems as though I dwell excessively on *my* son's life and death, *my* feelings as a mother about his journey, it is because Michael stands as a symbol of *all* who have fallen from AIDS. My grief is your shared grief. My experiences are yours.

For AIDS is not just an ugly set of statistics that soar daily into astronomical numbers. AIDS is your brother, your sister, your husband, your wife, your child, your lover, your friend —and mine as well.

In *The AIDS Caregiver's Handbook,* Ted Eidson and his contributors have shared with all of us the lives of their brothers, lovers, and friends touched by AIDS. Interspersed with medical and psychological and practical how-tos are extraordinary stories of compassion, courage, and caring. They are called appropriately "Stories from the Front." They tell the truth of what it is like for the caregiver moving forward in the war against AIDS. They are personal stories of grace and gratitude. It's as if we count our days "Before AIDS" and "After AIDS." We are changed forever.

I wrote the following words, chronicling Michael's last days: "The human spirit is resilient. The human spirit *is* love. Each of us had hourly opportunities to question and to experience the intensity of our feelings and the validity of our beliefs. We were challenged in each moment to be the love, the absolute, no-holds-barred, unconditional love that Michael had asked for. We were forced again and again to stretch ourselves to the limit of endurance, to the limit of love as we know it."

The extraordinary people in *The AIDS Caregiver's Handbook* have indeed stretched themselves to the limit of love as we know it. I honor their contribution as I honor my son, and I celebrate with them in their continuing love as they reach out to others with this handbook.

May this book help, heal, bless, and benefit all who read it and all who experience it.

"You are safe. It's only change. Go forward in love."

SECTION I

MEDICAL ASPECTS

1

· AIDS 101 ·

CHARLES E. HALEY, M.D., M.S.

Charles E. Haley, M.D., M.S., has been the Chief Epidemiologist and Director of Communicable Diseases for Dallas County since 1984. Prior to that, he spent four years with the federal Centers for Disease Control where, as an Epidemic Intelligence Service Officer, he worked with Legionnaires disease, cholera, plague, encephalitis, and malaria. He received his Masters in Epidemiology at the University of Virginia and his Doctor of Medicine from Southwestern Medical School.

With the publication on June 5, 1981, of a report regarding five homosexual men who had an unusual type of pneumonia, the individual's relationship with others was changed forever. The report was published in the United States's Centers for Disease Control's Morbidity and Mortality Weekly Report, but the realization of the change did not become apparent until years later. The disease these young men had was Acquired Immune Deficiency Syndrome (AIDS). Since that report, enormous progress has been made in elucidating the nature of the virus that causes the syndrome, the ways to treat some of the complications, the epidemiology of the disease, and the modes of transmission; great strides have been made in the understanding of the disease and the virus, but no cure and no vaccine can yet be forecast.

Compared to other great epidemics of man, the progress against this epidemic is unparalleled.

Due to the long latency of the virus before the disease becomes evident, the disease penetrated far into society before it was recognized; and even when it was recognized, it was several years before decision makers became aware of the implications of the epidemic. As of 1991, the United States Public Health Service estimates that about one million Americans are already infected. In addition, more will become infected before a vaccine or a cure is ready, if ever.

▪ THE VIRUS ▪

AIDS is caused by a sexually transmitted virus known as the Human Immunodeficiency Virus (HIV) type I, which is transmitted through blood and semen. The virus belongs to a class of viruses known as retroviruses because of their unique ability to transcribe their genetic material (RNA) into DNA and actually insert that piece of DNA into the DNA of the host cell. Usually RNA is made from DNA, not vice versa: hence the name "retroviruses." The technology to deal with retroviruses is very new and is really a product of the research on cancer in the sixties and seventies. There are a number of different kinds of retroviruses, but the first human retrovirus was discovered in the late 1970s and named Human T-Leukemia Virus (HTLV, later known as HTLV-I). When the AIDS virus was first discovered, two groups found it almost simultaneously: The French named their virus Lymphadenopathy Associated Virus (LAV), while the Americans named theirs Human T-Cell Lymphotropic Virus Type III, or HTLV-III.

There are several properties that make HIV infections unique. First is the fact that the HIV genetic material (RNA) is actually integrated into the host cell's genetic material. This makes this kind of virus very ominous since it is doubtful that any kind of treatment can be developed to subsequently remove the viral genetic material. Also viruses with that property of "integration" often result in chronic neurological disease or cancer many years after infection.

Another major property of HIV is its uncanny ability to change its outer coat or "envelope protein." The molecular basis for this variation is uncertain, but it shares this property with other retroviruses. This variation in the envelope must be accounted for in developing a vaccine against AIDS and in testing for HIV.

To infect a person, HIV must enter the cells. To enter the cells, HIV must first attach itself to the outer membrane of a cell. Not all cells have receptors that allow HIV to attach; in fact, the variety of cells infected by HIV is very limited. The main class of cells infected by HIV are the "helper T-cells," or CD4 lymphocytes, which are a type of white cell responsible for orchestrating the immune response. When HIV wipes out a significant number of these cells, a person becomes susceptible to infection from other organisms.

Other cells that HIV can infect are the macrophages, which are amoeboid cells that scavenge the body for foreign matter. The consequence of infection of these cells is uncertain.

▪ THE DISEASE ▪

Once a person becomes infected with HIV, that person may develop any of a variety of manifestations. This disease is similar to many other infectious diseases in that there is a broad spectrum of host responses. Some persons become infected, develop an inability to fight off other infections, and die; for these people, we have a special name for their syndrome: AIDS. Others have the very same infection but have lesser degrees of immune suppression; but they do have weight loss, diarrhea, and other symptoms. For these people the name "AIDS-Related Complex" or "ARC" is often used. However, at any given time, most of the infected people are asymptomatic or only mildly symptomatic.

It really does not matter which "syndrome" a person has because a majority of infected people will suffer severe medical consequences as a result of the infection. Ten years after infection, more than 50 percent will develop AIDS without treatment. Some scientists estimate that 75 to 100 percent of the infected persons will develop AIDS after fifteen or twenty years of follow-up. Many HIV-infected persons develop a loss of intellect, or dementia. It is not clear what the origin of this dementia is, but some scientists believe that it is related to the HIV infection of the macrophages in the brain. What other syndromes may be associated with this virus (cancers, especially) are unknown.

Why some people develop AIDS and others do not is not clear. Numerous studies have looked at a number of potential cofactors, but the only cofactor thought to be important is time-since-infection: that is, the longer the time since initially infected with HIV, the more likely to develop AIDS. The mean time from infection to diagnosis of AIDS appears to be about ten years; some persons, especially infected children, get sicker much sooner, while others take longer.

Before 1987, from the time a person was diagnosed as having AIDS until death was a mean of about one year. Use of some of the newer antiviral drugs prolongs that time to more than thirty months. People with Kaposi's sarcoma (KS) and no other opportunistic infection may live longer.

The syndromes caused by HIV have no specific symptoms, so that diagnosing HIV infections and AIDS is based mainly on laboratory tests. In general, any symptom that persists—such as diarrhea, unintended weight loss, and swollen lymph nodes —could signify the presence of an HIV infection.

· THE TEST ·

Most of the laboratory tests that are available actually test for antibodies that a person's body makes in response to infection with HIV. Shortly after a person is infected, the body tries to fight off infection by making antibodies; production of these specific antibodies begins within a couple of weeks after infection but may not be detectable for four weeks to six months later. No laboratory test is perfect, but the available HIV-antibody tests yield very few false positive or false negative results, especially among individuals practicing high-risk behaviors (. . . unprotected sexual intercourse, needle sharing among IV-drug users); the predictive value of the tests is less among those not practicing high-risk behaviors.

Two main approaches have been used to assay for HIV antibodies: ELISA (enzyme-linked immunosorbent assay) and Western Blot. The newest ELISA tests that are being used now are much improved over the first-generation tests.

Tests that actually test for the virus are also available but are very expensive and suffer from many false negatives. These may be helpful in differentiating between true positives and false positives.

The information gained by HIV antibody testing can be psychologically damaging to an individual, but it is important medical information: A physician will consider a different set of diagnoses knowing someone has an HIV infection. In addition, infected persons should take sensible precautions to protect their health, including immunization against pneumococcal disease, annual immunization against influenza, and testing for tuberculosis. Infected persons are virtually certain to suffer some illnesses as a consequence of infection, so they should find a physician and get regular examinations and check levels of CD-4 lymphocytes.

Another sort of testing is also necessary. In patients with AIDS, specific tests are performed to diagnose the various infections or cancers they may have. These tests will vary with the specific problem.

■ TREATMENT ■

Treatment for AIDS and HIV infections is expensive and only marginally successful. Specific treatment for the opportunistic infections and cancers has varying success depending on the underlying condition of the patient and the disease. Currently, antiviral drugs that prolong the lives of HIV-infected people, such as azidothymidine (AZT), are available. Other drugs are being tested now and some may prove useful. It is unlikely that any drug will be found that will "cure" AIDS; probably the best that can be hoped for is a drug or a combination of drugs that will prolong the productive lives of infected people and produce minimal side effects.

■ TRANSMISSION ■

One of the things that is well understood about AIDS is its epidemiology. By 1983, numerous epidemiological studies had been performed that have sketched the epidemiology of the disease. One of the problems with this disease is that HIV is a virus of humans and does not readily infect other species; consequently, knowledge about how the virus is transmitted must be gained from studies of humans. However, it is highly unethical (and illegal) to deliberately expose people to such a deadly virus experimentally. For these and other reasons, an experimental approach to discovering how the disease is transmitted is not feasible. Therefore, we must rely on observing the virus and the disease as it exists in a human population: This process is called epidemiology. Through survey techniques, an epidemiologist will study infected persons and compare them to uninfected persons. From this comparison, the epidemiologist will observe differences between the infected and the uninfecteds, and from these observations of differences, will make inferences about how the disease is transmitted. In other words, this is an *inferential* approach rather than an *experimental* approach.

The problem with this inferential approach is that one cannot prove what does not occur. One can show very well how the disease is transmitted, but cannot show how it is not transmitted. The three main modes of transmission are by sexual intercourse, by direct inoculation of blood, and from infected mother to infant, perinatally. There are rare transmissions by other routes, but these are really variations of the above three routes.

Most of the cases in the United States represent sexual transmission, mostly among males who engage in sexual activities with other males (a broader group than just homosexual males). There is clear evidence for transmission among heterosexuals, both from male to female and from female to male. There has been one case report of transmission from female to female, sexually.

The second most common mode of spread is by direct inoculation among illicit drug users who share needles (again, a broader group than drug abusers). This is an especially acute problem in cities such as New York City and Newark. Other persons infected by direct inoculation include transfusion recipients, hemophiliacs, and health-care workers who suffer inadvertent needle-stick injuries.

Most of the infected children in the United States were infected perinatally, from infected mothers. Whether this transmission occurs in utero or during birth is unclear.

There are rare individuals infected by other routes. Several persons have been infected by artificial insemination; several by organ transplantation; and several laboratory workers have been infected by intense exposure to blood and body fluids. All of these represent unusual types of exposure.

Although epidemiology cannot "prove" that transmission cannot occur in other ways, the absence of certain observations can be reassuring. There have been *no* cases among the nonsexual household contacts in more than 200,000 AIDS cases; eleven separate studies have shown no transmission in households where there is an infected person; there have been no infections among children in contact with AIDS- or HIV-infected children.

Transmission by other routes is unlikely, and if it occurs at all, will not account for very many cases. AIDS and HIV infec-

tions are primarily spread by sexual intercourse, direct inoculation, and perinatally.

Several other points about the epidemiology need to be
considered. The proportion of persons with HIV infections who
subsequently develop AIDS is uncertain. After ten years of
follow-up, about 50 percent of infected men in a study in San
Francisco have developed AIDS; some people estimate that 100
percent of infected people will eventually develop AIDS.

The interval between infection and development of AIDS is
about eight to ten years on the average; some may develop AIDS
ten or fifteen years after infection.

Currently, it appears that most, if not all, HIV-infected persons are lifetime carriers of the virus. Whether any antiviral
treatment will alter the infectivity of an infected person is not yet
known.

▪ PREVENTION ▪

There are only three possible ways to prevent AIDS: a vaccine
to protect the uninfected, a curative treatment for infected persons, or the adoption of behaviors that will not spread the virus.
Due to the variability in the envelope proteins of the virus, and
due to the nature of this virus, no single, all-inclusive vaccine can
be expected soon, though several vaccines are being developed.
No treatment is likely to result in removal of the viral genetic
material from the host cell. The current treatments are not cures
but, rather, are palliative measures. If a "curative" treatment is
found, its use in public health would be limited by the inability
to identify infected persons early in the course of infection. In
addition, to be effective, the treatment should be given to infected persons and their sexual contacts; but it is probably not
feasible to find all infected persons until late in the course of their
infection.

This leaves only a behavioral approach, at least for the foreseeable future. In the 1930s, this behavioral approach was called

"social prophylaxis"; now it is called "safer sex." The effectiveness of the behavioral approach is difficult to measure, but there seem to have been large behavioral changes among gay men since 1983.

Safer sex is really a simple concept; unfortunately, the translation of the concept to actual behavior is highly complicated, probably because human behavior is complicated. Since the disease is transmitted by sexual intercourse with an infected person, then the safest sex is not to have intercourse with an infected person. How this translates into behavior is complicated by the fact that most infected persons do not know that they are infected, much less whether their partners are.

A safer-sex strategy is to limit the number of partners, preferably to one long-term partner who is HIV-antibody negative. Failing that, a person should choose a partner who is likely to have had few sexual partners. When it is not known whether a partner is infected, use condoms and spermicides, especially those containing nonoxynol-9. Condoms are effective barriers in other sexually transmitted diseases and are probably effective against AIDS, but only if they are used properly.

Once safer sex is defined, the next problem is to carry that message to persons who are potentially at risk and to get them to adopt the safer behaviors. One only need look at the experience of smoking and cancer to see that this is no easy, or highly successful, task. With AIDS, the fear of the syndrome is great enough that many persons are willing to accept the safer behaviors.

But this is only part of the problem. In addition to reaching the people practicing high-risk sexual behavior, there is the problem of having to stop the spread of AIDS among illicit intravenous drug users, who often share infected needles. The virus is spread by injecting the blood of an infected person into the veins of another, who may in turn pass the virus to a sexual partner, or, in the case of a woman, an unborn child. The IV-drug user, living on the fringes of society, is difficult to contact. Once contact is established, one may find that the fear of AIDS is overshadowed by the drug user's very real, immediate needs. A user who needs a fix is not finicky about the cleanliness of needles; a person who needs money to buy a fix is not too finicky about safe-sex prostitution.

Since behavior is a highly complicated matter, a multifaceted approach will probably reach the greatest number of persons. For some to adopt safer sexual behaviors, all that is needed is some mass-media attention about AIDS. For others with compulsive sexual behaviors, participation in Sex Addicts Anonymous (SA) or intensive psychotherapy may be necessary, approaches generally outside the realm of public health. For many others, some amount of personalized or group counseling will help motivate a behavior change.

One method of making an impact on a person's behavior, in as short a time as possible, is to provide counseling in association with HIV testing. This seems to be an effective and efficient means of encouraging behavioral change.

2

∎ AIDS 201 ∎

COMPILED BY BRADY ALLEN, M.D.

Brady Allen, M.D., graduated summa cum laude from the University of Texas, Austin, in 1975 and went on to graduate fourth in his class from Southwestern Medical School, Dallas, Texas. He completed his internship and residency in Internal Medicine at the Yale-New Haven Hospital, New Haven, Connecticut, in 1982. Since then, Dr. Allen has operated a general practice in Internal Medicine in Dallas, while holding associate professorships in Internal Medicine at Baylor University Medical Center and Clinical Medicine at Southwestern Medical School.

Editor's notes: In talking with volunteers, AIDS or ARC patients, and their families, one becomes aware of the continuing confusion that surrounds a patient regarding his or her medical situation. Often none of the caregivers know what disease or diseases the patient has. AIDS itself is not a specific ailment in itself; rather, it is definitive of a number of illnesses. Knowing what the specific disease is allows a caregiver to have an idea what to expect of and from the patient. Recognizing the symptoms of the patient's disease allows the caregiver to be on the alert for changes in his or her condition, positive or negative. Often caregivers have been able to assist the attending physician by spotting a new symptom in their PWA's disease in time for the physician to arrest the new disease before it becomes life-threatening. In such instances, the caregiver did not have to know more than "This symptom isn't typical of pneumonia," for instance, in order to call in the experts.

The medications surrounding AIDS and ARC are equally confusing. The names are often unpronounceable and are sometimes referred to by brand names or initials. Often a caregiver will need to discuss medications with various physicians in order to let each know what the other has already prescribed, to let the attending physician know of adverse reactions to a particular drug, and so on. Knowing the names of the more common medications allows clearer communications and better patient care.

Because AIDS and ARC are diverse, not every ailment, symptom, and disease can be covered in charts such as those that follow. What is covered is what Dr. Allen recognized as the most common and frequent diseases, symptoms, or medications. The survival rates given in the second chart are generalized from Dr. Allen's and other physicians' *personal* observations; they are not meant to be "official" in any way. They are included as milestones rather than tombstones. Medical progress is being made daily in each of the diseases, which means that even as this book is read, the average survival rates will have increased.

Finally, the charts deal only with medical treatments presently approved by the FDA. Experimental medications are excluded as being neither widely available nor medically predictable.

The charts presented following page 17 are designed to be quick reference sources, only. They are not meant to be used diagnostically, prescriptively, or prophetically.

▪ **BIBLIOGRAPHY** ▪

Bach, M. C., Bagwell, S. P., Knapp, N. P., et al. "9-(1,3-dihy-droxy-2-proproxymethyl) guanine for cytomegalovirus infections in patients with the acquired immunodeficiency syndrome," in *Annals of Internal Medicine*, 1985, 103: 381–382.

Felsenstein, D., D'Amico, D. J., Hirsch, M. S., et al. "Treatment of cytomegalovirus retinitis with 9-[2-hydroxy-1(hydroxymethyl) ethoxymethyl] guanine," in *Annals of Internal Medicine*, 1985, 103: 377–380.

Golden, J. A., Sjoerdsma, A., Santi, D. V. "*Pneumocystis carinii* pneumonia treated with a-difluoro-methylornithine: A prospective study among patients with the acquired immunodeficiency syndrome," in *Western Journal of Medicine*, 1984, 141: 613–623.

Groopman, J. E., Gottlieb, M. S., Goodman, J., et al. "Recombinant a-2 interferon therapy for Kaposi's sarcoma associated with the acquired immunodeficiency syndrome," in *Annals of Internal Medicine*, 1984, 100: 671–676.

Haverkos, H. W. "Assessment of therapy for *Pneumocystis carinii* pnuemonia," in *American Journal of Medicine*, 1984; 76: 501–508.

Hawkins, C. C., Gold, J. W. M., Whimbey, E., et al. "*Mycobacterium avium* complex infections in patients with acquired immunodeficiency syndrome," in *Annals of Internal Medicine*, 1986, 105: 184–188.

Kaplan, L., Volberding, P. A., Abrams, D. A. "Treatment of Kaposi's sarcoma (KS) in acquired immunodeficiency syndrome (AIDS) with alternating vincristine-vinblastine," in *Cancer Treatment Report*, 1986, 70: 1121–1122.

Klein, R. S., Harris, C. A., Small, C. B., et al. "Oral candidiasis in high-risk patients as the initial manifestations of the acquired immunodeficiency syndrome," in *New England Journal of Medicine*, 1984, 311: 354–358.

Krown, S. E., Real, F. X., Cunningham-Rundles, S., et al. "Preliminary observations on the effect of recombinant leukocyte A interferon in homosexual men with Kaposi's sarcoma," in *New England Journal of Medicine*, 1983, 308: 1071–1076.

Laubenstein, L. J., Krigel, R. L., Odajnyk, C. M., et al. "Treatment of epidemic Kaposi's sarcoma with etoposide or a combination of doxorubicin, bleomycin, and vinblastine," in *Journal of Clinical Oncology*, 1984, 2: 1115–1120.

Leoung, G. S., Mills, J., Hopewell, P. C., et al. "Dapsone-trimethoprim for *Pneumocystis carinii* pneumonia in the acquired immunodeficiency syndrome," in *Annals of Internal Medicine,* 1986, 105: 45–48.

Levine, A. M., Gill, P., Meyer, P., et al. "Retrovirus and malignant lymphoma in homosexual men," in *Journal of the American Medical Association,* 1985, 254: 1921.

Luft, B. J., Brooks, R. G., Conley, F. K., et al. "Toxoplasmic encephalitis in patients with the acquired immunodeficiency syndrome," in *Journal of the American Medical Association,* 1984, 252: 913–915.

Protnoy, D., Whiteside, M. E., Buckley, E., et al. "Treatment of intestinal cryptosporidiosis with spiramycin," in *Annals of Internal Medicine,* 1984, 102: 202.

Quintiliani, R., Ownes, N. J., Quercia, R. A., et al. "Treatment and prevention of cropharyngeal candidiasis," in *American Journal of Medicine,* 1984, 77: 44–47.

Sands, M., Kron, M. A., Brown, R. B. "Pentamidine: A review," in *Review of Infectious Disease,* 1985, 7: 625–634.

Siegal, F. P., Lopez, C., Hammer, G. S., et al. "Severe acquired immunodeficiency in male homosexuals, manifested by chronic perianal ulcerative herpes simplex lesions," in *New England Journal of Medicine,* 1981, 305: 1439–1444.

Small, C. B., Harris, C. A., Friedland, G. H., et al. "The treatment of *Pneumocystis carinii* pneumonia in the acquired immunodeficiency syndrome," in *Archives of Internal Medicine,* 1985, 145: 837–840.

Soave, R., Danner, R. L., Honig, C. L., et al. "Cryptosporidiosis in homosexual men," in *Annals of Internal Medicine,* 1985, 102: 593.

"Update: Treatment of cryptosporidiosis in patients with acquired immunodeficiency syndrome (AIDS)," in *Morbidity and Mortality Weekly Report* from the Centers for Disease Control, 1984, 23: 117–119.

Volberding, P. A., Abrams, D. I., Conant, M., et al. "Vinblastine therapy for Kaposi's sarcoma in the acquired immunodeficiency syndrome," in *Annals of Internal Medicine,* 1985, 103: 333–338.

Wharton, M., Coleman, D. L., Fitz, G., et al. "Trimethoprim-sulfamethooxazole or pentamidine for *Pnuemocystis carinii* pneumonia in the acquired immunodeficiency syndrome," in *Annals of Internal Medicine,* 1986, 105: 37–44.

Wong, B., Gold, J. W. M., Brown, A. E., et al. "Central nervous system toxoplasmosis in homosexual men and parenteral drug abusers," in *Annals of Internal Medicine,* 1984, 100: 36–42.

Yarchoan, R., Weinhold, K. J., Lyerly, K. H. "Administration of 3'-azido-3'-deoxythymidine, an inhibitor of HTLV-III/LAV replication to patients with AIDS or AIDS-related complex," in *Lancet,* 1986, 1: 575–580.

Ziegler, J. L., Beckstead, J. A., Volberding, P. A., et al. "Non-Hodgkin's lymphoma in 90 homosexual men: Relation to generalized lymphadenopathy and the acquired immunodeficiency syndrome," in *New England Journal of Medicine,* 1984, 331: 565.

Zuger, A., Louie, E., Holzman, R. S., et al. "Cryptococcal disease in patients with the acquired immunodeficiency syndrome," in *Annals of Internal Medicine,* 1986, 104: 234–240.

AIDS CHART ONE

(by system/organ)

Affected Body System	Signs and Symptoms

I. Nervous System

    A. brain & spinal cord

headache, fever, neck stiffness, seizures
photophobia
paralyses of face, arms, legs
loss of coordination/balance
involuntary movement of
    extremities
slurred or garbled speech
depression, agitation
decreased ability to perform
    routine tasks
decreased intellectual capacity
labile emotions
loss of judgment
loss of memory
inability to concentrate
double vision, vertigo
inappropriate social behavior

Specific Diseases	Treatment

I. Meningitis

   A. cryptococcus neoformans   amphotericin B
                                            fluconazole

   B. atypical tuberculosis   combination of 5 drugs:
       (aTB)   ethambutol
                                            clofazimine
                                            rifampin
                                            ciprofloxacin
                                            amikacin

   C. histoplasmosis   amphotericin B

   D. candida albicans   amphotericin B
                                              fluconazole

   E. Human   AZT (also called zidovidine or
       Immunodeficiency Virus   ZVD)
       (HIV)   possibly ddI or ddC

II. central nervous system mass
    lesions

   A. toxoplasma gondii   sulfa & pyrimethamine
                                            clindamycin & pyrimethamine

Affected Body System	Signs and Symptoms
I. Nervous System *cont.*	
B. peripheral nerves	numbness, tingling, burning, and pain of extremities (usually lower legs and feet)
C. eyes	photophobia (sensitivity to light) visual loss blurry vision scotomata (bright spots in visual field) eye pain
II. Cardiopulmonary System	
A. lungs	fever (usually greater than 100 degrees) dry cough shortness of breath chest pain (especially on deep breath)

Specific Diseases	Treatment
B. cryptococcoma	amphotericin B fluconazole
C. primary lymphoma	whole brain radiation
D. progressive multifocal leukoencephalopathy (PML)	no available treatment
E. Kaposi's sarcoma (KS) (rare)	chemo/immunotherapy
III. peripheral neuropathy	
A. cytomegalovirus (CMV)	DHPG may be helpful
B. HIV	no effective treatment
IV. retinitis	
A. CMV	DHPG phosphonoformate
B. candida albicans	amphotericin B fluconazole
C. toxoplasma gondii	sulfa & pyrimethamine clindamycin & pyrimethamine

I. pnuemonia	
A. pneumocystis carinii (PCP)	sulfa & trimethoprim (oral or IV) pentamidine (IV or aerosolized) trimethoprim & dapsone clindamycin & primaquine should add steroids if pO_2 is less than 70

II. Cardiopulmonary System *cont.*

    B.   heart   chest pain
                                               rapid heartbeat
                                               fainting
                                               shortness of breath

Specific Diseases	Treatment
B. mycobacterium tuberculosis (typical TB)	combination of 3 drugs: isoniazid rifampin ethambutol
C. atypical TB	combination of 5 drugs: ethambutol clofazimine rifampin ciprofloxacin amikacin
D. CMV	DHPG (effective in 30–50% of cases)
E. cryptococcus neoformans	amphotericin B fluconazole
F. histoplasmosis	amphotericin B
G. coccidiomycosis	amphotericin B
H. Kaposi's sarcoma (KS)	combination chemotherapy
I. lymphoma	combination chemotherapy

II. myocardial infiltration

A. atypical TB	same as for atypical TB above
B. CMV	no effective treatment
C. histoplasmosis	amphotericin B
D. cryptococcus neoformans	same as above

II. Cardiopulmonary System *cont.*

III. Gastrointestinal System

    A. mouth

loss of taste
change in taste
dry mouth
sore tongue or gums
nonhealing mouth ulcers
white coating on tongue and
    cheeks
lumps on gums, soft or hard
    palate
excessive bleeding of gums

    B. esophagus and
        stomach

pain on swallowing
severe heartburn
chest pain
weight loss
loss of appetite
upper abdominal pain
intermittent nausea

Specific Diseases	Treatment
E. Kaposi's sarcoma	same as above
F. lymphoma	chemotherapy

I. mucositis/glossitis

A. candida albicans (thrush)	nystatin mouthwash or lozenges clotrimazole troches ketoconazole fluconazole
B. hairy leukoplakia	no effective treatment
C. nonhealing herpes simplex	acyclovir phosphonoformate

II. mass lesions of mouth

A. KS	chemo/immunotherapy
B. histoplasmosis	amphotericin B
C. diffuse B-cell non-Hodgkin's lymphomas	combination chemotherapy

III. esophagitis and gastritis

A. candida albicans	fluconazole ketoconazole amphotericin B

III. Gastrointestinal System *cont.*

    C. large and small
       intestines

chronic diarrhea (with blood or
  mucous)
weight loss (usually greater than
  10 pounds)
lower abdominal pain
nausea (with occasional
  vomiting)
fever
night sweats
severe fatigue

Specific Diseases	Treatment
B. herpes simplex	acyclovir (Zovirax)
C. CMV	DHPG
D. diffuse non-Hodgkin's lymphoma of stomach	combination chemotherapy
III. gastroenteritis/colitis	
A. CMV	DHPG
B. cryptosporidium	no effective treatment
C. atypical TB	combination of 5 drugs: ethambutol clofazimine rifampin ciprofloxacin amikacin
D. isospora belli	sulfa & trimethoprim
E. HIV	AZT may be of benefit
F. microsporidia	no effective treatment
IV. mass lesions of large and small intestines	
A. KS	chemo/immunotherapy
B. non-Hodgkin's lymphoma	combination chemotherapy

III. Gastrointestinal System *cont.*

    D. liver

yellow eyes
nausea
vomiting
fever
chronic fatigue
tea-colored urine
light-colored stools
right-sided upper abdominal pain

    E. rectum

rectal pain
rectal discharge
rectal bleeding
rectal ulcers
fecal incontinence
fever

V. hepatitis

    A. atypical TB

        combination of 5 drugs:
           ethambutol
           clofazimine
           rifampin
           ciprofloxacin
           amikacin

    B. cryptococcus neoformans   amphotericin B
           fluconazole

    C. CMV   DHPG

VI. mass lesions of liver

    A. KS   chemo/immunotherapy

    B. non-Hodgkin's   combination chemotherapy
       lymphoma

VII. proctitis

    A. nonhealing herpes   acyclovir
       simplex   phosphonoformate

    B. CMV   DHPG

III. Gastrointestinal System *cont.*

IV. Skin

flat or raised purple lesions
easy bruisability
red scaly rash of face
unexplained recurrent hives
diffuse infection of hair follicles
reactivation of dormant warts
nonhealing ulcers or blisters
multiple tiny bleeding spots
    under the skin

Specific Diseases	Treatment

C. atypical TB	combination of 5 drugs:
	  ethambutol
	  clofazimine
	  rifampin
	  ciprofloxacin
	  amikacin

D. KS	combination chemotherapy
E. lymphoma	combination chemotherapy

I. tumors

A. KS	chemo/immunotherapy

II. common rashes (not
diagnostic of AIDS but
suggestive of HIV activation)

A. recurrent folliculitis	antibiotics (oral or topical) dermatological soaps
B. seborrheic dermatitis	steroid creams medicated shampoo (tar-based) Nizoral cream
C. herpes zoster (localized or disseminated)	high-dose acyclovir
D. chronic eczema	steroid creams
E. recurring yeast dermatitis	clotrimazole ointment ketoconazole fluconazole

Affected Body System	Signs and Symptoms

IV. Skin *cont.*

V. Immune System

    A. lymph nodes and spleen

fever
fatigue
night sweats
swollen glands (in neck and
    under arms)

Specific Diseases	Treatment
F. molloscum contagiosum (chronic and recurrent)	excision
G. nonhealing herpes simplex	acyclovir
H. tinea cruris or corporis	clotrimazole ointment ketoconazole ointment griseofulvin

I. tumors

    A. KS — chemo/immunotherapy

    B. diffuse B-cell non-Hodgkin's lymphoma — combination chemotherapy

II. infections

    A. atypical TB — combination of 5 drugs:
        ethambutol
        clofazimine
        rifampin
        ciprofloxacin
        amikacin

    B. histoplasmosis — amphotericin B

    C. coccidiomycosis — amphotericin B

    D. cryptococcus neoformans — amphotericin B / fluconazole

    E. CMV (not diagnostic of AIDS) — DHPG

    F. HIV (lymphadenopathy syndrome) (not diagnostic of AIDS) — AZT

AIDS CHART TWO

Disease (Disease Type)	Symptoms
B-cell lymphomas, high-grade diffuse [cancer]	fever, night sweats, weight loss, bone pain, loss of appetite, swollen lymph glands
candida albicans: esophagitis or disseminated: liver, lungs, brain, blood, bone marrow [fungus]	Primary: pain on swallowing, weight loss, nausea, loss of appetite Secondary: headache, fatigue
coccidiomycosis	fever, malaise, weight loss
cryptococcus neoformans (cryptococcosis): disseminated (bone marrow, liver, blood) or meningitis	Primary: fever, headache, nausea, confusion Secondary: seizures, paralysis, irrational behavior, night sweats, weight loss

Treatment	Prognosis	Major Side Effects
various chemotherapeutic regimens employing 4–6 different agents, all highly toxic		Depends on the therapy used. See side effects for KS for examples.

60% response rate with a 50–60% relapse rate; 30% complete remission. Average survival 4–6 months.

Treatment	Major Side Effects
ketoconazole: 200–400mg., orally, once daily (probably should be treated indefinitely due to high rate of relapse)	nausea, headache, skin rash, dry mouth, hepatitis, enlarged breasts
fluconazole: 100–200mg. once daily	skin rash, elevated liver functions
amphotericin B: 0.2–0.3mg./kg. daily I.V. for 2 weeks (for disseminated or severe disease not responsive to ketoconazole)	chills, fever, headache, flushing, nausea, vomiting, hepatitis, kidney failure, anemia, low potassium

90–95% cure rate with 60–70% relapse rate. Average survival is 6–8 months after diagnosis.

Treatment	Major Side Effects
amphotericin B	fever, chills, nausea

6–8 months

Treatment	Major Side Effects
amphotericin B: 0.6mg./kg./day I.V. for 8–12 weeks for a total dose of 1500–2000mg.	chills, fever, headache, flushing, nausea, vomiting, hepatitis, kidney failure, anemia, low potassium
fluconazole: 400mg. initially, then 200mg. daily for 2–3 months	skin rash, elevated liver functions

Disease (Disease Type)	Symptoms
cryptococcus neoformans *cont.*	
cryptosporidium (cryptosporidiosis) [parasite]	severe diarrhea, fever, weight loss, fatigue, abdominal cramps
cytomegalovirus (CMV): retinitis, gastroenteritis, or disseminated (bone marrow & brain) [virus]	Primary: fever, chills, loss of vision, scotomata, diarrhea, weight loss Secondary: headache, confusion, muscle aches, cough, shortness of breath
HIV encephalopathy [virus]	headache, dementia, incoordination, seizures, paralysis, loss of memory, brief attention span, poor judgment, visual disturbances
HIV wasting syndrome [virus]	weight loss of 10% of body weight, night sweats, fever, fatigue, diarrhea
herpes simplex II: chronic mucocutaneous infection lasting more than 1 month (unhealing genital or rectal herpes) or esophagitis [virus]	rectal pain, rectal discharge, fecal urgency, fever, swollen glands in groin, pain on swallowing

Treatment	Major Side Effects
Prognosis	

Survival of acute infection is about 30%. Average survival after treatment is about 6–8 months. High relapse rate, about 80%, after stopping amphotericin. Patients need close follow-up and need to be treated prophylactically with fluconazole at 100–200mg. daily indefinitely.

no treatment available

Average survival is 2–4 months.

DHPG (9–1, 3dihydroxy–2propocymethyl guanine): 5mg./kg. of bodyweight I.V. every 12 hrs. for 14 days, then 6mg./kg. I.V. once daily 7 days/wk. continued indefinitely	low white blood cell count, low platelet count, skin rash

80% response rate with 100% relapse rate after drug is stopped. Average survival is 6–8 months.

azidothymidine (AZT) (also called zidovidine or ZVD): 100mg. orally every 4 hrs.	headache, nausea, decreased appetite, diarrhea, anemia, low white blood count, insomnia, body-aches

30–50% response rate. Average survival is 4–6 months.

AZT: 100mg. every 4 hrs.

40–50% response rate. Average survival is 3–6 months.

acyclovir: 200mg. orally every 4 hrs. for 7–10 days, then twice daily indefinitely; or if oral dose not effective, may give 10mg./kg. I.V. every 8 hrs. until lesions healed	nausea, low white blood count, mild kidney failure

Disease (Disease Type)	Symptoms
herpes simplex II *cont.*	
histoplasma capsulatum: (histoplasmosis) disseminated: mouth, GI track, liver, bone marrow, brain [fungus]	Primary: fever, chills, night sweats, weight loss Secondary: cough, joint aches, swollen lymph glands
isospora belli [parasite]	diarrhea, fever, weight loss
Kaposi's sarcoma (KS) [cancer]	purple spots on skin or gums, swollen glands, fatigue, night sweats, fever, weight loss

Treatment	Major Side Effects
Prognosis	

90–100% response rate. Average survival is 18 months, though herpes itself is not fatal.

Treatment	Major Side Effects
amphotericin B: 0.6mg./kg./day I.V. for a total dose of 2 grams	chills, fever, headache, flushing, nausea, vomiting, hepatitis, kidney failure, anemia, low potassium
followed by	
ketoconazole: 400–600mg. orally per day to prevent recurrence	nausea, headache, skin rash, dry mouth, hepatitis, enlarged breasts
or	
amphotericin: 50–100mg. once or twice weekly to prevent recurrence	same as above

60% response rate with a greater than 60% relapse rate. Average survival after treatment is 6–9 months.

Treatment	Major Side Effects
sulfa/trimethoprim: 1 double-strength tablet twice daily for 6–8 weeks (Bactrim or Septra)	depressed appetite, nausea, vomiting, skin rash, hepatitis, kidney failure, fever, anemia, low white count, low platelet count

80–90% response rate with a 30% relapse rate. Survival rate is unknown at this time.

Treatment	Major Side Effects
vinblastine: variable dosage	nausea, vomiting, loss of appetite, pain and tingling of hands and feet, anemia, low white blood count
vincristine	peripheral neuropathy
alpha interferon: high dose	flulike illness symptoms, nasal congestion, muscle weakness, elevated liver functions, neutropenia

Kaposi's sarcoma (KS) *cont.*

Disease (Disease Type)	Symptoms
mycobacterium avium complex (atypical TB, MAI, MAC, intracellulare) [bacteria]	fever, fatigue, weight loss, cough, diarrhea, swollen lymph glands, night sweats

Treatment	Prognosis	Major Side Effects
leomycin		fever, nausea, pulmonary fibrosis
ombination of one or more of the bove agents plus others not listed		same as above but more toxic

0–40% partial remission rate with frequent relapses and a 1–3% complete remission rate. Average survival time is 18 months. Most experts do ot treat KS unless there is a cosmetic or obstructive complication or unless here is evidence of internal organ involvement. The chemotherapeutic gents listed are very toxic and further depress cellular immunity, thereby ncreasing the risk of opportunistic infections.

ombination of the following 5 drugs:

Treatment	Major Side Effects
thambutol: 12–20mg./kg. orally nce daily	dermatitis, joint pains, nausea, itching, headache, dizziness, dislocation, decreased vision
lofazimine: 100mg. orally once aily	skin discoloration, dry skin, nausea, vomiting
mikacin: 15mg./kg. per day IM ntramuscular injection) or I.V. divided twice daily	kidney failure, decreased hearing, muscular weakness
ifampin: 600mg. orally once daily	hepatitis, abdominal pain, nausea, diarrhea, dizziness, incoordination, confusion, inability to concentrate

Disease (Disease Type)	Symptoms
mycobacterium avium complex *cont.*	
mycrobacterium tuberculosis extrapulmonary sites	
pneumocystis carinii pneumonia (PCP) [protozoa]	Primary: fever, dry cough, shortness of breath Secondary: fatigue, weight loss, headache

Treatment	Prognosis	Major Side Effects
ciprofloxacin: 500mg. twice daily		nausea, skin rash

40–60% of patients report an improvement in symptoms. These drugs are usually not curative. Average survival is 4–6 months.

Treatment	Major Side Effects
isoniazid: 300mg. orally once daily	burning and pain in feet, hepatitis, arthritis, anemia, dizziness, stupor, loss of coordination, optic neuritis
ethambutol: as above	same as above
rifampin: as above	same as above
pyranzinamide: 20–30mg./kg. orally divided in 4 doses	hepatitis, gout, arthralgias, loss of appetite, nausea, vomiting, pain on urination

Must treat for at least 12 months and perhaps indefinitely.

Treatment	Major Side Effects
sulfa/trimethoprim: 15–20mg./kg. divided every 6 hrs., orally (2 double-strength tablets) or I.V. (4 ampules) for 14 to 21 days (Bactrim or Septra)	Depressed appetite, nausea, vomiting, skin rash, hepatitis, kidney failure, fever, anemia, low platelet count
pentamidine isoethionate: 4mg./kg. I.V. once daily for 14 to 21 days. For mild PCP, you may use aerosolized pentamidine: 600mg. once daily for 21 days.	low blood pressure, low blood sugar (during infusion), fever, nausea, vomiting, diarrhea, loss of taste, skin rash, kidney failure, anemia, low white count, low platelet count, decreased appetite, diabetes (usually after more than 2 wks. therapy), pancreatitis

pneumocystis carinii pneumonia *cont.*

salmonellosis (disseminated)	fever, chills, cramping, bloating, diar-rhea
toxoplasma gondii (toxoplasmosis) [protozoa]	Primary: headache, fever, visual dis-turbances Secondary: paralysis, seizures, cranial nerve palsies

Treatment Prognosis	Major Side Effects
trimethoprim: 15–20mg./kg. divided every 6 hrs., IM or orally	depressed appetite, nausea, vomiting, skin rash, hepatitis, kidney failure, fever, anemia, low white count, low platelet count+
+	
dapsone: 100mg. orally once daily	loss of appetite, nausea, vomiting, headache, insomnia, fever, blurry vision, hemolytic anemia in patients with G6PD deficiency
+	
corticosteroids: 40mg./day if oxygen level is below 70	

70–80% cure rate with 20% chance of relapse. Prophylaxis with daily sulfa/ trimethoprim (one double-strength tablet daily) or aerosolized pentamidine (300mg. once monthly) may be effective in preventing reccurence. Cure rate declines to 15–20% if patient requires ventilatory support. Average survival rate prior to availability of AZT was about 36 weeks; survival rate average with AZT is 21 months.

Treatment Prognosis	Major Side Effects
ampicillin or trimethoprim-sulfa or ciprofloxacin	rash, fever, nausea
unknown	

Treatment Prognosis	Major Side Effects
sulfadiazine: 1–1.5gr. orally 4 times daily	fever, nausea, vomiting, headache, skin rash, hepatitis, low white count, low platelet count, kidney failure
+	+
pyrimethamine: 100mg. initial dose followed by 50–75mg. orally once daily	anemia, low white count, low platelet count
+	+
folinic acid: 10–30mg. once daily. Treatment should continue forever. After the first 6 weeks, pyrimethamine may be reduced to 25mg.	none
If patient is allergic to sulfa, may substitute clindamycin 1200–1800mg. (I.V. or orally) daily for 6 wks.	

60% response rate with average survival after diagnosis of 6–8 months.

3

·NUTRITION·
AND THE
IMMUNE SYSTEM

ALAN I. HAMILL, D.O.

Alan I. Hamill, D. O., graduated from the Texas College of Osteopathic Medicine after the completion of undergraduate work at the University of Pennsylvania and graduate studies at the University of Connecticut. He is currently in private practice in Dallas, Texas, emphasizing self-responsibility in the creation of health or illness. In addition to traditional medicine, he offers preventive/nutritional counseling, acupuncture, osteopathic, and various alternative treatments that enhance one's innate capacity to heal one's self.

■ HOW THE IMMUNE ■
SYSTEM OPERATES

Human immunity is comprised of many structures with diverse functions. Among these are included our skin, the mucous membranes of the nose, saliva, stomach acid, and the varied cellular components. AIDS impairs that part of the immune system that is called "cellular." This includes a complex and sophisticated collection of cells that can recognize other cellular components as being either "same" or "foreign." This distinction protects the body against invasion and destruction. These "foreign" cells or collection of cells can be as diverse as viruses, bacteria, parasites, and fungi, or many other nonself materials such as chemicals. In all cases these nonself invaders are labeled "antigens" (against self).

White blood cells are the primary component of the cellular immune system. One type of white blood cell, the macrophage, is capable of destroying antigens directly. Such cells also serve the function of "presenting" or marking organisms for destruction. Other white blood cells, the lymphocytes, act indirectly. There are two types of lymphocytes: T-cells (which are programmed in the thymus gland) and B-cells (which mature in the bone marrow).

T-cells recognize a foreign invader and then influence other cells to help attack the antigen. Their intermediary role gives rise to the term "cell-mediated immunity." T-cells are subdivided into many varieties. Of greatest importance here are T-4 helper cells and T-8 suppressor cells. T-4 helper cells stimulate either B-cells or other T-cells into activity. T-8 suppressor cells inhibit cellular immune activity. In essence, they say, "Enough is enough!" One of the hallmarks of impaired immunity is a reversal of the normal ratio of T-4 to T-8 cells. Normally, there are almost twice as many helper cells as suppressor cells. In immune-compromised people, there are more suppressor cells than helper cells, causing the immune system to shut down instead of gearing up to fight infection.

B-cells are involved in "humoral immunity." After B-cells leave the bone marrow, they rest in lymph organs: glands (also called "nodes") and the spleen. Their specific function is to filter blood and fight infection. As blood is being filtered, B-cells recognize an antigen, enlarge, and split into "plasma cells," which, in turn, produce antibodies. The antibodies are protein molecules that are released into the bloodstream, where they seek out copies of the original antigens that spurred their production. Upon recognition, the antibodies adhere to the surfaces of the antigens, forming special complexes that act as markers. Scavenger cells, called "phagocytes," locate the marked foreign material and destroy it by consuming it.

Another component in cellular immunity is the natural killer or NK-cell, which may be a form of T-cell. It is active in devouring cells such as cancer cells that are dysfunctional and reproducing out of control.

There is a very sophisticated balance between all of these components. For instance, macrophages, after ingesting an antigen, will alert certain T-cells to release a substance that informs the B-cells to produce antibodies for the original antigen. A disruption at any phase of the system may affect the entire immune-response process.

Both T-cells and B-cells have "memories" and will recognize an antigen that they have encountered before. Upon subsequent exposure to a foreign invader, circulating cells will alert the body to mount a massive production of the particular antibody needed to counter the antigen invasion. This is what is involved in skin testing. A common antigen is applied to the skin, and if the immune system is functioning properly, cells are called to the region to fight the antigen invasion, causing redness and swelling. In a patient whose immune system has been compromised, this will not happen; cells do *not* rally to fight the invasion.

▪ HOW NUTRIENTS ▪ DIRECTLY AFFECT IMMUNITY

Now that you have a general understanding about what the cellular immune system is and how it works, we will explore how the various vitamins, trace elements, and other nutrients work to help create or bolster it. There has been a great deal of interest in the past decade in nutrition (witness the profitable health-food industry); but many people have no idea what it is all about. They buy whichever vitamins and supplements happen to be popular at the time without any idea as to what they do or how they work. They are unaware that a combination of two supplements may either enhance or nullify one another.

The purpose of this section is to acquaint you with the basic nutrients: what they are, what they do, how they interact, and where they can be found organically. Supplementation guidelines are given, as well.

First, it is important to understand that we often eat foods that are stripped of their natural nutrients during processing. Instead of nutrients, we eat chemicals added to enhance flavor or prolong shelf life. These chemicals can inhibit our body's immune system. Additionally, antibiotics and hormones that are fed to livestock to counter disease and encourage growth may have deleterious effects on the human body; and pollutants in our air and water further weaken our defenses. Because of these factors, most of us do not get all the necessary nutrients we need from our everyday diet to provide the greatest immunity possible.

▪ GENERAL DIET ▪

Initially, one must realize that a practical, balanced diet is the essential foundation upon which any nutritional program should be based. There is a great amount of disagreement regarding the various percentages of the primary food groups—carbohydrates, fats, and proteins—that would comprise an optimum regimen. There are many diets and plans to investigate, any of which (with a little common sense and a modicum of effort) yield impressive results.

The main thing is to avoid chemically enhanced foods and "fast" foods. These have been processed to the degree that they are robbed of essential vitamins and minerals. Also, they are frequently prepared in harmful fats, which they absorb. Concentrate on fresh vegetables, preferably raw or lightly steamed to retain natural nutrients. Vegetables provide minerals, vitamins, some protein, and fiber. Be sure to thoroughly wash or peel the vegetables when appropriate to remove the residue of any chemicals that might have been utilized to assist growth.

Eating fresh vegetables also allows one to focus on seasonal foods. This helps give the body specific foods throughout the year that are beneficial to the body's cycle. It also helps to prevent the development of possible allergies to specific foods from repetitive usage. There is ample evidence that rotating foods helps prevent development of food allergies, while repetitive consumption leads to allergic sensitivity.

Carbohydrates are excellent sources of energy for the body. They are composed of differing natural sugars that can be readily utilized during the energy drain of disease states. They are a very efficient, economical source of ready energy and are best consumed in the form of complex starches such as potatoes, rice, grains, fruits, and vegetables. These starches are broken down into the sugars that supply the energy (calories) our bodies need to function.

Complex starches are excellent sources of nutrition and should be emphasized over proteins as a staple in our diet. They provide a steady, utilizable source of sugar that nourishes our body rather than depleting it as, for instance, sugar cane does. The sugars in complex carbohydrates are released slowly into the system, allowing for proper digestion, usage, and storage. Cane sugar is not fully absorbed and remains in the bloodstream. This creates two problems. First, fungi and viruses feed on this excess sugar, which helps them grow and multiply. Second, the pancreas is strained to release exaggerated amounts of insulin to metabolize the excess sugars quickly. This depletes the body's readily available stores of energy, causing a "crash," a feeling of overexertion, or "the sugar blues."

Complex carbohydrates also provide some vitamins, minerals, and fiber, depending on the specific source. Whole-wheat breads are an excellent source of carbohydrates, nutrients, and fiber. They enhance digestion while providing needed nutrients.

Legumes such as peas, beans, and certain nuts, in addition

to their high levels of carbohydrates, are also able to provide our total needs for protein. Regrettably, most of our protein is attained from animal products that are contaminated with chemicals and saturated with harmful fats.

Americans eat much more protein than they require. Most adults require only 25 to 40 grams of protein daily. An individual's average protein needs can be estimated by multiplying his or her weight in pounds by a factor of 0.28. The result is read in grams of protein needed per day. Note, however, that chronically ill people require 25 to 50 percent more protein than healthy individuals.

Excess proteins shorten life. There are definite indications that excess proteins, particularly from animal by-products, can inhibit the immune system and lead to several problems, among which are cancer, heart disease, obesity, and kidney disease. In addition, such foods usually take more energy to digest. They are very inefficient sources of energy. Red meats are the worst, due to chemical saturation and harmful fats. Chicken is better, but it is generally so polluted with estrogens (to enhance growth) and antibodies (to prevent disease) that it, too, should be limited in one's diet. Fish is a very good source of protein and provides oils that help protect against heart disease.

The fats that are present in meat products, fried foods, butter, and two of the major oils (palm and coconut) used in processed foods are very hard on the heart. Fats have been linked to the development of several cancers and various autoimmune diseases, such as systemic lupus. Fats in excess impair the immune system and should be reduced in everyone's intake.

Conversely, some proper fats are essential to maintain the integrity of cell walls. They are also essential for the formation of a class of molecule called "prostaglandins," which is an intermediary in the inflammatory process. Beneficial fats are found in seeds, nuts, and fish oils. Fish oils are more readily available and more beneficial when obtained from fish itself rather than from capsules. For cooking, cold-pressed virgin olive oil is a good substitute for most polyunsaturated oils, which by virtue of being processed are not optimum sources of appropriate fats. However, polyunsaturated oils are better than those derived from animal by-products.

There are specific components of proteins that are essential to health and immunity; and if a totally vegetarian diet is chosen, be careful to learn how to combine nuts, beans (legumes), grains, seeds, and vegetables to allow for the proper complement necessary for optimum health. There are several cookbooks readily available for education in this realm and many have charts listing the protein, carbohydrate, and fat contents of various foods.

In summary, lots of fresh vegetables, fruits, and complex carbohydrates are a good basis for a diet to enhance health and immunity. Utilize fat-laden protein products only for indulgence or celebration on rare occasions.

■ VITAMINS ■

Vitamins are naturally occurring nutrients that the body cannot produce and that are needed in minute quantities to enable various bodily functions to occur. They are essential to maintain immunity, and a shortage can lead to severe disease. The rationale for vitamin supplementation is twofold. First, the habits of processing and cooking depletes foods of their natural vitamins. Second, during illness or chronic vitamin deficiency, one generally is unable to replenish the vitamin stores by using an average American diet.

The "recommended daily allowance" (i.e., RDA) of vitamins was developed during wartime to establish quantities necessary to afford a mass populace (the armed forces) the *minimal* nutritional requirements. In essence, this allows for minimal health. We are interested in maximizing health, not merely subsisting. Therefore, some of the suggestions that follow may indicate seemingly excessive quantities of certain nutrients. When megadoses of vitamins are recommended, it is to replenish or supply maximum possibility of full health and immunity. This does not mean "more is better." In fact, in certain cases, excessive vitamins can be detrimental. Megadoses are recommended only where prior research has indicated their usefulness with minimal side effects. One theory suggests that only synthetic vitamins should be megadosed. The logic of the argument states that natural supplements have cofactors and enzymes that assist their assimilation by the body. These characteristics are not found in the synthetics. Thus, megadoses of the synthetics may be required in order to provide enough to be assimilated in an amount equal to the natural vitamins.

In explaining benefits, immune enhancement (either direct or indirect) will be the primary emphasis: Vitamins do a lot more for the body than just enhance immunity.

VITAMIN A

Vitamin A has been shown to have a direct influence on immunity, with deficiencies leading to infection in the respiratory system and digestive tract. The body's ability to make antibodies and to maintain cell-mediated immunity is compromised with vitamin A deficiency. One study (Weiner, p. 99) showed that normal postsurgical immune suppression could be lessened with vitamin A megadoses. Vitamin A has also been found to have anticancer properties and may be useful in preventing the immune suppression seen in chronic stress cases (Weiner, p. 100). Vitamin A is formed from beta carotene. In certain aspects of immune enhancement, ingesting beta carotene has been shown to be more effective than ingesting vitamin A.

Green and yellow fruits and vegetables are good sources of vitamin A. In particular, apricots, cantaloupes, sweet potatoes, carrots, spinach, and parsley supply vitamin A. Also, it can be found in liver, eggs, dairy products, and fish liver oil. Doses of this vitamin in the range of 10,000 to 50,000 IU (International Units) per day should be easily tolerated. It is normally stated that 50,000 units of vitamin A daily may lead to toxicity. The patients in the Cahen experiment, however, received much larger doses for seven days with no apparent toxicity. Acutely, toxicity manifests as vomiting, headaches, dizziness, and blurred vision. Ingesting 100,000 IU per day, chronic changes such as dry itchy skin, weight loss, hair loss, and liver damage with jaundice may occur. An appropriate maintenance dose is 25,000 units per day.

Vitamin E and zinc have been found to act synergistically (helpfully) with vitamin A, but cortisol (steroid) antagonizes it (Kutsky, p. 181). Vitamin A levels directly influence vitamin C: a deficiency of vitamin A can decrease vitamin C's ability to function effectively (Kutsky, p. 181).

B VITAMINS

Thiamine or vitamin B_1 is mainly associated with carbohydrate metabolism and nerve conduction. It has some minimal effects on the immune system (Weiner, p. 101). Vitamin B is found primarily in cereals, wheat germ, rice, soy flour, yeast, fruit, animal products, beans, and peas.

Riboflavin or vitamin B_2 helps maintain mucosal barriers that are so essential in maintaining our bodies' defenses. Mucous membranes are those moist linings of the mouth and nose, lungs, digestive, vaginal, and urinary tracts that are our first defenses against disease. They are barriers that must be penetrated before infection can take place, and their integrity is essential for maximum functioning of the immune system. Riboflavin also enhances lymph-organ size and antibody responses (Weiner, p. 101). B_2 supplementation is necessary with antibiotic treatments, liver disease, fevers, and traumatic stress (Kutsky, p. 225). Organ meat (like liver), dairy products, and brewer's yeast provide high quantities of B_2. Corn, califlower, beans, and saffron are also good sources. The normal supplement is 50 mg. up to several grams. It is essentially nontoxic in humans.

Vitamin B_6 or pyrodoxine provides important immune functions in humans. Deficiencies have been shown to lead to impairment of both cell-mediated and hormonal immunity (Weiner, p. 102). Pyrodoxine is also critical to the maintenance of mucous membranes. It is important to know that pyrodoxine is antagonized by the antituberculosis drug, isoniazide, as well as penicillamine, which is an antiinflammatory, antirheumatic drug (not to be confused with penicillin). Both of these medications are sometimes used in AIDS treatments. Vitamin B_6 is synergistic with B_2 and niacin in maintaining skin integrity and may be involved with vitamin B_1 for nerve tissue maintenance (Kutsky, p. 240). It must be replaced in conditions of irradiation, high-protein diets, and stress. High concentrations are found in liver, herring, salmon, yeast, nuts, wheat germ, brown rice, and blackstrap molasses. Other sources are bananas, avocados, apples, pears, carrots, tomatoes, and onions. Daily supplements are 50 to 200 mg. Excess amounts can lead to toxicity.

Vitamin B_{12}, or cyano cobalamin, functions mainly in the synthesis of red blood cells, proteins, and lipids, and is important in nerve-cell maintenance. Deficiency of B_{12} alone is extremely rare, and, therefore, its effects on immunity are questionable. Some studies have implicated it in the building of the immune system's T- and B-cells, as well as the phagocytic (killing) and bacterial responses of immune cells (Weiner, p. 103). One important fact is that vitamin B_{12} is antagonized by vitamin C and must be replenished if vitamin C therapy is instituted. It is mainly obtained in animal products: Vegetarians must supplement their diet with B_{12}. It is also found in egg yolks, fish, and dairy products to a limited degree. Usual supplementation is 50 to 100 micrograms per day. Toxicity is rare.

VITAMIN C

Ascorbic acid, vitamin C, is one of the rare instances where studies have been performed to show the actual benefits of megadoses, rather than simply to prove the damaging effects of deficiencies. The studies are extremely controversial, without conclusive arguments from either side of the debate. Linus Pauling was the first person to popularize the belief that megadoses of vitamin C could counter various viral illnesses, ranging from the common cold to influenza. Most researchers have found some reduction in the intensity of viral infections with vitamin C supplementation, but few use the massive quantities called for by Dr. Pauling. The mechanism of action is unknown, but it is known that vitamin C can enhance phagocyte migration and killing functions, as well as wound healing (Beisel, p. 55). Dr. Pauling and a colleague, Dr. Cameron, have reported success with some cancer patients given 10 grams of vitamin C per day, but these results have been disputed. Dr. Robert Cathcart has reported success with some AIDS patients given huge doses of vitamin C, some by IV. Dr. Cathcart suggests increasing daily dosages up to the point where bowel intolerance (diarrhea) is reached, then decreasing the dosage by 10 percent. Since this treatment requires massive quantities of vitamin C, which may be harmful, it is essential that the protocol be followed only under the supervision of a practiced physician.

Other points of interest are the antistress properties of vitamin C, as well as its function as an antioxidant, which helps protect against the creation of free radicals (see explanation of free radicals under Vitamin E, page 57). It is also valuable in the detoxifying actions of heavy metal pollutants (lead, cobalt) and of pesticides (Kutsky, p. 252).

Aspirin (specifically acetosalicylic acid, not acetaminophen or Tylenol) causes loss of vitamin C, and the constant use of aspirin to combat fevers in AIDS patients can lead to a vitamin C reduction (Weiner, p. 106). Vitamin C in large doses can inactivate B_{12} and cause kidney stones, diarrhea, and other problems. Corticosteroids and copper antagonize vitamin C, while vitamins A and E, zinc, and iron are synergistic to it. Vitamin C is found in citrus products, rose hips, green peppers, parsley, papaya, and strawberries. Conditions requiring extra vitamin C are stress, infections, allergies, high-protein diets, and trauma. Ascorbic acid should be taken in quantities starting at 1 gram per day up to bowel tolerance. Because it is rapidly excreted by the body, it should be divided into several doses throughout the day for maximum efficiency. If the acidity of some preparations upsets the digestive tract, this effect can be mitigated by ingesting a buffered form.

VITAMIN D

Vitamin D is produced by our bodies and is stored in the fat tissue. Sunlight is required for its activation. It may actually be *immunosuppressive* in excess and toxicity occurs at relatively low doses, so supplementation should be avoided. It is essential for calcium and phosphorus metabolism and is generally available in adequate quantities in the most average of American diets. It is obtained from liver oils, egg yolk, sea food, milk products, and some grains (enriched).

VITAMIN E

Vitamin E is noted for its antioxidant properties. Membranes are susceptible to substances called "free radicals," which are produced in a chemical process called oxidation. Vitamin E helps counter the effects of free radicals resultant from oxidation and is called an "antioxidant." This is especially important in protecting against some cancers. For instance, substances called "nitrates," which are found in foods such as barbequed meats, can be metabolized into cancer-producing nitrosamines. The antioxidant properties of vitamin E protect against this. It also helps retard breakdown of red blood cells by the same process.

Regarding immunity, vitamin E can enhance resistance and protect macrophages from the products of oxidation secondary to their bactericidal actions (Beisel, p. 56). This requires doses of two to twenty times the minimal daily requirements. Megadoses can be quite toxic and immunosuppressive, so quantities must be regulated (Beisel, p. 56). Selenium (to be discussed under trace minerals on page 61) acts synergistically as an antioxidant, as does vitamin A. Iron antagonizes vitamin E. Although vitamin E is fat-soluble, it is excreted fairly rapidly and is removed from foods during processing; so supplementation may be important for maintaining a level of this vital substance. It is found in wheat germ, crude vegetables, grain oils, soybeans, and yeast. It is required in excess for areas of high pollution and for diets laden with processed foods or polyunsaturated fats (Kutsky, p. 200). Supplements range from 100 to 1,200 IU per day.

▪ THE ACIDS ▪

Folic acid is essential for immunity. Deficiencies lead to impaired cell-mediated and humoral immunity (Beisel, p. 55). It is also essential for B_{12} absorption, and deficiency leads to a very debilitating anemia. One of the major causes of folic acid deficiency is alcoholism. Synergists are vitamins C, B_{12}, pantothenic acid, iron, and copper. Folic acid is found in green vegetables (spinach), organ meats, milk, yeast, legumes, peanuts, tuna, and whole grains. It needs to be supplemented in illnesses, gastrointestinal diseases (which inhibit absorption), diarrhea, antibiotic therapy, Hodgkin's disease, and in cases of anemia (which is quite prevalent as a side effect of many drugs used to combat AIDS).

Pantothenic acid is essential as a part of coenzyme A, which is instrumental in energy metabolism and antibody synthesis (Kutsky, p. 286). It acts synergistically with other B vitamins as well as folic acid, niacin, and biotin. Deficiencies are rare in an American diet. It is found in organ meats, brewer's yeast, legumes, wheat germ, and eggs, as well as in many other foods. Toxicity is rare and dosages range from 50 mg. up. It has been noted as being a necessary supplement in stress, arthritis, illness, depression, and burning foot syndrome (Kutsky, p. 286). The latter is a discouraging condition seen with some AIDS patients. This supplementation is generally attained with diet alone.

▪ MINERALS ▪

More than 99 percent of the body is composed of the inert compounds carbon, hydrogen, oxygen, and nitrogen. These passive chemicals exist in quietude until acted upon by a small group of catalytic minerals that activate enzymes to catalyze reactions to form compounds. These activating minerals are called "trace minerals" because a mere trace amount will allow a reaction. Conversely, even a minute reduction of one of them will inhibit or reduce necessary functional activities. Hence, they are of a critical nature and cannot be overlooked in the maintenance of immunity. They are often removed in food processing and can be depleted by chemicals ingested in treated foods or polluted air and water.

COPPER

Copper is a plentiful mineral that is essential for bodily functioning. Although critical in immunity, blood formation, chemical respiration, and as an antioxidant, *it can be harmful in excessive quantities.* It is present in most foods and can be consumed in excess due to its presence in cooking utensils, beverage containers, or soft water. High concentrations are found in oysters, soybeans, nuts, wheat germ, yeast, corn oil, and bone meal. Excess consumption can interfere with absorption of iron and zinc. In a true deficit, supplementation would be 2 to 5 mg. daily.

MAGNESIUM

Magnesium shortage or depletion in man has not been shown to have an effect on immunity. Ironically, long-term magnesium deficiency in lab animals has been shown to lead to increased white cells and eventually to leukemia and thymus malignancy. The deficiency has also been shown to lead to a release of histamine, a mediator in allergic reactions, and reduced response to normal antigens. (Beisel, p. 56). Magnesium is critical to normal bodily functions for the synthesis of proteins and various vitamins, hormones, and enzymes. Its chief antagonist is calcium. People taking calcium supplements should consider adding a magnesium supplement in a 1:1 ratio. Many supplements are sold in a 2:1 ratio, which is counterproductive.

True magnesium deficiency is rare in a standard American diet, but excess phosphorus in meats, preserved foods, and soft drinks may lead to decreased magnesium stores. Phosphorus, like calcium, can interfere or compete with magnesium during absorption. Nuts, wheat germ, blackstrap molasses, soybeans, and brewer's yeast are good sources of magnesium. Daily supplementation, if necessary, should be in the range of 300 to 500 mg.

IRON

Iron deficiency is one of the more common problems with AIDS patients. Often, due to lack of absorption from diarrhea or anemia secondary to malnutrition and drug side effects, the AIDS patient is depleted of iron. A deficiency of iron can lead to multiple immune dysfunctions, including atrophy of lymphoid tissues, decreased sensitivity to antigens, and defective cellular response to infectious assaults (Beisel, p. 56).

It is important to realize that too much iron can also be deleterious to health. Iron levels can be checked by a simple blood test. Excess iron can antagonize zinc, which is also an important immune enhancer. Iron supplements must be monitored carefully. Excess iron ingestion during times of infection can give the infectious agents the iron that they need for survival and actually feed the infecting organism. It is important only to take supplements when needed. However, iron is important for transport of oxygen, and proper levels must be maintained. Therefore, it is imperative to periodically check iron levels in malnourished or anemic people.

In malnourished people, there can be a deficit of the proteins that carry iron in the blood; so there can be excess iron in the blood, iron not bound to proteins, which is then available as food for infectious organisms. Therefore, iron replacement in protein-malnourished individuals is especially delicate. Excess iron has also been implicated in cancer development (Weiner).

Natural foods are the best source for a balanced iron intake. Iron is found in high concentrations in shellfish, organ meats, spinach, nuts, wheat germ, bran, and brewer's yeast. Vegetarian diets are generally low in iron. Cast-iron pots and pans used for cooking release iron but can lead to toxicity. The ferrous (Fe^{2+}) form is more readily absorbed than the ferric (Fe^{3+}) form. Supplementation is usually 15 to 50 mg. per day. Do not take supplements of iron unless under educated guidance.

ZINC

Zinc is another mineral that is essential for optimum immunity, yet may be detrimental in excess. It is critical for proper functioning of cell-mediated immunity; and deficiency can reduce the number of mature T-cells, interfere with response to antigens, and delay proper wound healing (Beisel, p. 56). On the other hand, excess zinc has been found to inhibit immune functions. In particular, the normal functioning of neutrophils and macrophages are impaired by excess zinc. This mineral probably achieves its influence via the many enzymatic reactions that it helps catalyze. Zinc is essential for carbohydrate metabolism and is instrumental in the maintenance of prostate integrity.

Infectious agents feed on excess zinc as they do excess iron. Consequently, it is probably best to utilize foods for supplementation rather than synthetics: eat oysters, sunflower and pumpkin seeds, cheese, wheat germ, bran, brewer's yeast, beef, and liver. Boiling vegetables (instead of gently steaming) removes needed zinc. If supplementation is utilized, 15 to 50 mg. per day is a standard range.

SELENIUM

Selenium has been found to have an immune-enhancing effect when administered experimentally in excess of normal dietary intake. It was found to produce enhanced antibody formation to vaccines (Crary). This is thought to be further enhanced by vitamin E in combination with selenium. It is also shown in lab animals to be an effective inhibitor of cancer (Weiner, p. 115). It is a very effective antioxidant and is useful in countering the effects of heavy metal poisoning (such as cadmium and mercury). However, like iron, too much of a good thing can be harmful and very large doses can be toxic. Therefore, one must be cautious when supplementing. Foods high in selenium are seafood, wheat germ, brown rice, bran, barley, brewer's yeast, liver, kidney, Brazil nuts, cashews, and peanuts. The supplemental range is 10 to 100 mg. Please exercise caution.

▪ CONCLUSION ▪

One of the easiest and seemingly most sane ways to provide optimum dietary nutrition and immune enhancement is to eat a balanced, fresh diet of vegetables, fruit, complex carbohydrates, low protein, and low fats. Supplement this with a natural multivitamin with trace minerals. It isn't necessary to buy many bottles of individual vitamins: You would only be paying extra for packaging, inert ingredients, filler, complexity, and annoyance. I also recommend 3,000 mg. of vitamin C with breakfast, lunch, and dinner. After this, all else must be individual. Chronically ill people will require an additional 25 to 50 percent of protein. People suffering from thrush (candida) might benefit from acidophilus (which resupplies a natural component of our digestive tract) or an increase in daily bran. One tablespoon of bran daily has been proven to enhance bowel function and regularity.

Before starting a nutritional program, it is imperative that you find a truly knowledgeable person to consult. This can be a health practitioner, dietitian, health-food store worker or friend. Please refrain from believing that any single diet or supplement is *the answer.* There are no exclusive answers; however, there are ways of eating nourishing foods while avoiding harmful substances. This advice carries over into the realm of supplements, as well. There are herbs, teas, clays, diets, homeopathic drops, flower essences, and any number of equally diverse, confusing, and potentially helpful items to ingest. The diversity correlates with the diversity of symptoms and the people experiencing them. Find a system that feels best to you, that fits your life and philosophy. Then, stick with it long enough to see the results. This may take weeks. If you flip from one regimen to another, you will never know what may be helping and what may be hurting.

▪ BIBLIOGRAPHY ▪

Badgley, Laurence, M.D. *Healing AIDS Naturally: Natural Therapies for the Immune System.* San Bruno, CA: Human Energy Press, 1987.

Beisel, William R., et al. "Single-Nutrient Effects of Immunologic Functions." *Journal of the American Medical Association (JAMA),* January 2, 1981, vol 245, no. 1, pp. 53–58.

Crary, E.G., G. Smyrna, and M.F. McCardy. "Potential Applications for High Dose Antioxidants." *Medical Hypotheses,* 1984, 13: 77–98.

Kutsky, Roman J. *Handbook of Vitamins, Minerals and Hormones.* New York: Van Nostrand Reinhold Co., 1981.

Weiner, Michael A. *Maximum Immunity.* Boston, MA: Houghton Mifflin Co., 1986.

4

· AIDS 301: · ALTERNATIVE TREATMENTS

ALAN I. HAMILL, D.O.

Alan I. Hamill, D.O., graduated from the Texas College of Osteopathic Medicine after the completion of undergraduate work at the University of Pennsylvania and graduate studies at the University of Connecticut. He is currently in private practice in Dallas, Texas, emphasizing self-responsibility in the creation of health or illness. In addition to traditional medicine, he offers preventive/nutritional counseling, acupuncture, osteopathic treatment, and various alternative treatments that enhance one's innate capacity to heal one's self.

· INTRODUCTION ·

There are a number of treatment techniques that are available alternatives and/or adjuncts to traditional American medical therapeutics. Many of these techniques rely on the awareness that there must be an integration and balancing of the mind, body, and spirit in order for total healing to take place. These alternatives range from purely mental disciplines (such as meditation and guided imagery) through the spectrum of physical modalities (such as therapeutic massage and osteopathic medicine).

Any of the treatments discussed in this chapter may be beneficial to some, but each will not be appropriate to everyone. One must explore the options and experiment to find those treatments that suit one's personality as well as one's physical maladies. It is very important not to shift from treatment to treatment or practitioner to practitioner. One must allow sufficient time to see results. The conditions of Being that have culminated in the development of AIDS have taken time to manifest, and they may require an equal amount of time to cure. Traditional medicine will help in supporting the fight against acute attacks of opportunistic diseases, such as *Pneumocystis carinii* pneumonia. However, many believe that much more is necessary in order to aid one in regaining the Balance needed to allow one to overcome a state of weakened immunity.

It is very helpful if one can find a truly holistic physician or health practitioner, a person who is well versed in Western medicine and alternative treatments. Such a doctor can help one understand the available options, establish an appropriate regimen, and monitor traditional treatments.

The object of nontraditional treatments is to maintain health, a concept thought to be more important than simply fighting disease after it has manifested. If body, mind, and spirit can be sufficiently fortified, disease will not be able to penetrate one's defenses. For this reason, much of this chapter is relevant to caregiver and PWA alike: to *maintain* the caregiver's health and to *regain* the PWA's or PWARC's health.

This will be a cursory introduction with the purpose of acquainting you with the most frequently used alternative treatments for AIDS and ARC. There are a number of references listed in the Appendix so that you may pursue whatever treatment holds interest for you.

▪ PHYSICAL TREATMENTS ▪

Initially, let us begin with those treatments considered to be physical or hands-on techniques. One of the biggest problems with AIDS patients is that they become divorced from their bodies: "It" is discussed, and the AIDS patient wants to escape "it" or hide from "it." A PWA or PWARC is touched less, and often becomes rigid and defensive in both attitude and body. The physical treatments create relaxation, aid in the awareness of the body and its dynamic tensions, and are designed to enhance the body's inherent capacity to heal itself.

▪ OSTEOPATHIC ▪

The belief in the body's own healing capabilities is the basis of osteopathic medicine. A Doctor of Osteopathy (D.O.) has been trained and licensed like a Medical Doctor (M.D.) in traditional medicine. In addition, he will receive special training in the musculoskeletal system (muscle, bones, connective tissue) and in techniques to manipulate the body to remove the tensions that inhibit the normal flow of blood, lymph, or neuroenergy. For example, if there is excessive tension in a particular bodily region, the muscles may become taut and rigid, and clamp down on the arteries, veins, and lymph channels running through and around them. The flow of nutrients and the removal of toxins from the area is lessened. Utilizing specific techniques of manipulation, an osteopathic physical can relax the tensions, release the blockages, and help restore normal functioning.

▪ CHIROPRACTIC ▪

Chiropractors are trained to adjust joints in the body with the goal of restoring normal bodily functioning. Emphasis is placed on the proper alignment of the spinal column due to the simple truth that all of the nerve-impulse messages to and from the brain must exit and enter through the column.

Chiropractic treatments are very beneficial in relieving body aches and pains, as well as in helping to restore normal functioning and structural integrity to the body. Though chiropractors are not trained or licensed in traditional medicine, many have explored other methods of treatment and can help in a variety of ways. They see healing as maintaining the body in concert with nature; and many are well versed in the more "natural" forms of therapeutics.

■ THERAPEUTIC MASSAGE ■

Massage treatments can be very therapeutic and may be an excellent means of reducing tension and learning more about the body. There are many different techniques of massage, but they all have in common the goal of focusing on physical tension and reducing it by working with varying amounts of pressure or touch. Because it takes energy for the body to maintain tension and muscular tightness (actually a contraction), when the tension is released, energy is freed to be used elsewhere in the body. By removing these muscular tensions, one has more energy to focus on healing.

■ ROLFING ■

A form of deep tissue manipulation that is related to massage is Rolfing. Developed by Ida Rolf, it is based on the theory that a body that is out of alignment is constantly fighting the forces of gravity just to maintain its integrity. This lack of alignment can be the result of physical or emotional posture. The trained Rolfer will work in a systematic manner in order to restore proper alignment and release tensions in the muscular system. This usually requires ten sessions.

There is some belief among Rolfers that there may be inherent "memories" of prior traumas that can be released along with muscular tension. For instance, a particular emotional trauma may have created a specific muscular tightening of the abdomen; and when the abdominal musculature is released via Rolfing, a subconscious memory of that incident may surface, allowing one to work through whatever residual sentiments may have been retained. When the emotion that originally caused the muscular tightening is worked through and released, the physical manifestation is not likely to reappear. If one can find a Rolfer who emphasizes this aspect of the process, the beneficial results are even greater.

▪ FELDENKRAIS ▪

Moshe Feldenkrais developed a technique of "Awareness Through Movement," wherein he postulated that one's movement is as individual as one's personality. By studying movement and posture and working to improve them, awareness of the personality structure is enhanced and changed. His technique is taught through a series of exercises performed while lying on the floor, so that normal gravitational considerations may be ignored. The exercises are designed to create a new sense of awareness of the body and its movement, an awareness of the body's state of being and health at any time.

Feldenkrais developed a one-on-one manipulative treatment called "functional integration," as well as individual exercises that can be taught by trained Feldenkrais practitioners to help one attain awareness of self through movement on an ongoing basis.

▪ ALEXANDER ▪

F. Matthias Alexander developed a technique of postural awareness after having studied his own problems of voice loss when performing as a Shakespearean actor. While studying himself in front of a mirror, he noticed that *thinking* of speaking caused a muscular contraction in his throat. He realized that thinking of motion resulted in contractions and bodily responses that were habitual but not necessarily beneficial. Furthermore, he conjectured that movement was learned, not merely reflexive. If one learned movement, then one could unlearn and relearn correct movements. Like Feldenkrais, he asserted that without mental awareness, the body cannot change. He also knew that the movement of one part of the body affects the entire body. Seeing movement as learned habits that can be relearned with proper study and mental awareness, he created a system of true mind-body discipline that can be of inestimable value to those suffering from bodily afflictions. One learns an entirely new awareness and control of mind over body. The techniques of awareness taught by this method can work in all aspects of Being and wellness, far beyond their applicability to physical bodily movement.

▪ APPLIED KINESIOLOGY ▪

Kinesiology is a system of studying muscular imbalances. Dr. George Goodheart, a chiropractor, discovered that many muscle spasms and tightness were caused by those muscles overcompensating for weakened muscles on the opposite side of the body. Combining this awareness with the Eastern philosophy of energy flow (discussed under Oriental Therapies), he developed a system of muscle testing and treatment that balances muscular tensions. These techniques have also been used to test for food allergies. The theory is that allergic substances weaken the muscles and beneficial substances strengthen them. Some practitioners even utilize muscle testing to verify the effectiveness of medicinal treatments.

▪ ORIENTAL THERAPIES ▪

There are several therapies that are traditional Oriental practices now being utilized by Western practitioners due to their successful application. These therapies are based on the fundamental

Oriental belief that the life force, or "chi" (pronounced "key"), flows through the body along very specific, circumscribed, invisible channels called "meridians." In a healthy individual, these forces are balanced evenly between what is known as yin and yang energies. The maintenance of this balance between opposing yin and yang forces is the goal of all Oriental treatments, indeed of most Oriental philosophies.

The yin and yang forces can roughly be divided as follows:

Yin	Yang
Earth	Heaven
Passive	Active
Contractive	Expansive
Dark	Light
Negative	Positive
Inner	Outer
Female	Male
etc.	etc.

It is very important to understand that these are conceptual and not concrete forms, relative rather than absolute.

The body is divided into yin and yang, also. The hollow organs, such as intestines and stomach, are considered yang, and the solid organs, such as liver and lungs, are considered yin. Each meridian relates to one of the organs, and diseases in the organs will be reflected in the increase or decrease of energy flow along the meridian. Likewise, if a meridian is overly stimulated or depleted, the disturbance will be reflected in the appropriate organs. There are very specific patterns of movements between the various meridians, and sophisticated treatments have been developed over many centuries based on these movements. They can be correlated to times of the day, seasons of the year, mutation of the elements of earth, wind, fire, and water, and many other systems of relatedness.

Imbalances within the system can be detected in a variety of diagnostic manners. All of the techniques that follow aim at restoring normal balance so that the yin and yang are in harmony and optimum health is restored, concurrent with a balanced flow of energy along all the meridians.

■ ACUPUNCTURE AND ACUPRESSURE ■

In acupuncture, needles are inserted at specific points along the meridians in order to balance the energy flows to either enhance weakened meridians or reduce overstimulated ones. In acupressure (or "shiatsu"), finger pressure is used instead of needles. Either can be a very beneficial aid in helping one restore balance in the face of illness, based on the assumption that balanced energies restore health and the capacity of the body to ward off disease. In AIDS patients, it may allow the restoration of certain strengths that have been lost due to the debilitating illness. It can be used comfortably in concert with traditional Western medicine.

As a word of warning, one may be better off with practitioners who have been trained in traditional Oriental diagnostic techniques as opposed to those who have studied "pain control"—someone who truly understands the concept of the body as a mass of energies that can be directed and balanced by their techniques as opposed to someone who is simply going to treat pain or disease with pat formulas. The best practitioners recognize disease as a result of imbalanced energy, and locate the source to treat. Others less indoctrinated in Oriental technique want to treat only the disease, leaving its root cause out of balance.

Acupuncture and acupressure are aids to rebalancing. But, as in all Oriental treatments, the patient must look at all aspects of his being—emotional, mental, physical, and spiritual—to determine why the energies are out of balance to begin with. This is why there is no clear division between Oriental philosophy and medicine as there is in the Western world; and this is why one should locate the traditionally trained practitioner to obtain the full benefits of treatment.

▪ MENTAL DISCIPLINES ▪

It is crucial to realize the power of thought in the healing process. It has been documented that emotional stress can deplete the immune system. Various studies have shown actual diminishment of immune-enhancing cells secondary to stress.

Thought is a form of energy in much the same manner that electricity is. It powers engines (our bodies), sends messages (words and sounds), and generates energy (heat secondary to activity and emotions). The law of conservation of energy is one of the basics of the universe. It states that energy is finite and constant. The energy that enters a system remains in that system until it is released as an equal amount of energy: The form of energy can be altered, but the quantity remains the same.

Thought, as a form of energy, can be transformed into sound, which, when transported through the air, can activate modern machines. The energy in the sound, literally, can trigger mechanisms to open gates, start recording devices, or turn off alarm clocks. This is the fundamental concept of the conservation of energy: It is never lost. The same thought forms which create sounds can be directed at our bodies, which are really only aggregates of energy, in order to alter them according to specific needs.

There are many methods of directing our thoughts in order to utilize mental energies to augment the healing process and to combat the debilitating effects of stress. Numerous articles, tapes, and books teach relaxation techniques, which are a fundamental prerequisite in calming the body or fortifying it and its defenses.

▪ BIOFEEDBACK ▪

One of the earliest modern techniques is called biofeedback. By use of a small machine that measures certain bodily characteristics, a tone will be emitted when a state of total relaxation has been reached.

Many different methods can be used to reach this state of relaxation. One utilizes an exercise wherein breathing is controlled consciously and directed at various parts of the body to draw air and energy into those areas and then to exhale tension from them. Another technique utilizes systematic tightening and relaxing of every muscle in the body from bottom to top, first to become aware of the difference between the feel of tense muscles (tension) and relaxed ones (relaxation), and second, to systematically create the state of physical relaxation.

▪ VISUALIZATION AND IMAGERY ▪

Some of the easiest and most accessible techniques utilize a method called "visualization." The Simontons of the Simonton Cancer Institute and many other practitioners have current books and articles on this subject drawn from their years of experience with cancer patients.

With eyes closed, one becomes completely relaxed, either by another method or, for example, by visualizing walking down a shaded stairway, becoming more and more relaxed as one descends into comforting darkness. Once relaxed, an image is brought to mind that may represent the desired change in any number of ways. Some people simply see themselves as being completely healthy. Others imagine the healing white blood cells as white knights charging forth, conquering the invading infections and visualizing the "bad guys" in full retreat. For those who may have trouble focusing clearly on an image, the suggestion is made to draw the desired image on paper to give it more substance and reality.

A number of tapes on visualization and imagery are listed in Appendix F. Many other tapes, books, and even classes are available through local metaphysical bookstores. Additionally, you will be able to find other sources through cancer specialists and psychotherapists. What was once thought of as a "bit strange" is now much more widely accepted. The practice of visualization or imagery is one of the most powerful healing techniques available today, and they are virtually cost-free when compared to the price of any other form of treatment. It should be used by all PWAs, PWARCs, and their caregivers daily.

▪ COLOR AND SOUND ▪

A distant cousin of visualization is color or sound therapy. It is thought that by using either the visualization of color or special machines that bathe a person in color, different moods or states of being can be created. For instance, studies have been performed that suggest the color red agitates, while pinks and pastel blues pacify.

Color therapy becomes more specific, though, by using exact wavelength colors to create desired effects on individual body areas. Additionally, various colors are representative of certain thought patterns that are tied to specific emotions. Thus, colors can be used to enhance certain thought patterns in order to create moods and emotions suitable for healing.

The effect of sound is obvious, and its utilization to enhance relaxation, visualization, or color therapy is immeasurable. However, there are a few practitioners who use sound in and of itself as a healing medium: Patricia Sun, for example. Vocal or instrumental sounds create certain vibrations that may create anything from simple relaxation to something akin to mild electrical currents, which are very pleasant and considered therapeutic.

There are a number of New Age cassette tapes and other meditation tapes that are available at record and bookstores everywhere. They range from electronic music to Eastern music to recorded sounds of whales, birds, or surf.

▪ MEDITATION ▪

Meditation and meditation tapes are another aspect of utilizing the mind to achieve relaxation, focus thoughts, and enhance health and immunity. Meditation is much easier than most people realize. It is simply clearing the mind of extraneous thoughts and focusing on something to elevate one's state of being. The object of focus may be a thought that is spoken aloud (sometimes called a "mantra"), an object that is seen (perhaps a flower, a spiritual guide, a candle, a "mandala," or even empty sky), or, in the "purer" forms of meditation, the void that is created with a complete openness to whatever may be. The key to this latter technique is not to focus on or grasp thoughts, but rather to observe them as they pass and then let them go.

Again, there are a number of excellent books available on meditation and the various techniques. There is no one *right way;* what works for you is correct.

• YOGA •

Yoga is a particularly beneficial blend of mind and body techniques. Through calming one's mind and relaxing one's body in coordinated fashion, a total state of relaxed awareness is reached.

There are many forms of yoga. The most common and popular is the school of Hatha Yoga. It employs various postures or "asanas" that have specific purposes. Each will either stimulate or calm particular parts of the body.

Initially, a series of breathing exercises is utilized to calm the mind and focus the energies on the task ahead. Then, in a systematic manner, each posture is attained through quiet contemplation of breath and physical stretching. The breath is utilized to ease the body into each asana. As an exhalation is performed, the body automatically releases tension (a physiological function) and further stretching into a posture can be achieved. As an inhalation is performed, visualization of life-giving energy is directed to the area of the stretch. As exhalation follows, greater flexibility and relaxation is achieved.

This is a gentle yet powerful tool for relaxation and bodily awareness. It is not only extremely healthy as a form of pure, gentle, rhythmic stretching exercise, it is also invaluable as a help in attaining an awareness of the dynamics of the musculoskeletal system and the power the mind has over the body.

▪ CONCLUSION ▪

Each of the alternative therapies that have been presented have myriad offshoots, and many have been combined so that it is difficult to determine where one ends and another begins. Curiously, it doesn't often matter. Unlike pharmaceutical treatments, none of these treatments clash if the spirit behind them is constant —that of balancing, harmony, and relaxation.

Medical practitioners have always recognized that their patient's attitude has a great deal to do with how fast the patient will recover or, conversely, how rapidly he will deteriorate. All the alternative treatments, at the very least, are directed toward creating the attitudes that enhance healing; and many people find that various of the alternatives have worked for them to unlock their own patterns of physical or mental energies in order to create active healing.

You can know the discipline that is appropriate for you simply because it feels correct and comfortable to you. Practice with it until you have been able to reach some stage of proficiency. At that point, you will better know if you need to add another dimension and what that alternative might be.

And, a final reminder: This chapter is written equally to the caregiver and to the PWA or PWARC. To be a caregiver on any level—lover or parent or medical practitioner—is stressful. Stress unchecked can lead to infirmity and illness. The disciplines discussed are extremely beneficial in bleeding off stress before it becomes debilitating. Too, they open untapped sources of energy, which allow us to continue performing the double duty inherent in the responsibilities of caring for another's health while maintaining our own.

▪ **BIBLIOGRAPHY** ▪

Badgley, Laurence, M.D. *Healing AIDS Naturally: Natural Thera-pies for the Immune System.* San Bruno, CA: Human Energy Press, 1987.

Inglis, Brian and Ruth West. *The Alternate Health Guide.* New York: Alfred A. Knopf, 1983.

Weiner, Michael A. *Maximum Immunity.* Boston, MA: Houghton Mifflin Co., 1986.

SECTION II

COPING, COUNSELING, AND CARING

5

·THE·
PSYCHOSOCIAL
ASPECTS OF AIDS

JACK HAMILTON, M.S.W., C.S.W.-A.C.P., AND VICKI L. MORRIS, R.N., M.S.W., L.P.C.

Jack Hamilton, M.S.W., C.S.W.-A.C.P., and Vicki L. Morris, R.N., M.S.W., L.P.C., have both been deeply involved with counseling PWAs, PWARCs, and their friends and relatives through the Oak Lawn Counseling Center and in private practice. Vicki received her M.S.W. from the University of Texas at Arlington; she is also a Master Practitioner of NLP (neurolinguistic programming). Jack has become increasingly involved in leading workshops and classes focusing on holistic approaches to wellness. After receiving his Masters in Social Work from the University of Oklahoma, he became a Counselor, and later Coordinator of Bereavement for Dallas Visiting Nurses Association.

▪ INTRODUCTION ▪

AIDS and ARC impact all who come into contact with them; and either can be devastating, not only to the person who is diagnosed, but also to lovers, spouses, family, and friends. This chapter provides an overview of the psychological and social challenges that are commonly faced from diagnosis onward by all concerned. Many of the experiences are similar to those faced in any serious illness; however, there are challenges unique to AIDS. How you and the PWA deal with these problems and issues will determine the quality of life that each of you will be able to maintain for the foreseeable future.

At the outset, it needs to be stated that not everyone will experience all of the issues that will be explored here, and many issues may arise that this chapter will not mention. Each AIDS or ARC situation is as unique as the people involved.

▪ DEFINING "PSYCHOSOCIAL" ▪

The term "psychosocial" is a combined word from "psychological" and "social"; and as the word suggests, it looks at the interactions between the two areas. The psychological (internal) challenges are often caused directly by social (external) changes; the reactions that one has psychologically will often be expressed socially. For example, in the case of a Person with AIDS (PWA) or ARC (PWARC) who has lost his or her job (social), s/he may have feelings about it (psychological) to such an extent that legal action (social) is taken.

Not only are the psychosocial issues interactive within a single individual, they are interactive among individuals. How you present your issues to your PWA or how s/he presents his or hers to you can have a direct bearing on the well-being of you both. The more you know about what the issues may be and how they can be handled, the healthier everyone will be.

▪ A WORD ABOUT HEALTH ▪

Throughout the ages, true health has been conceptualized as meaning more than only physical healing or the absence of illness. Before the modern age, healing encompassed total well-being, a balancing of a person emotionally, mentally, and spiritually, as well as physically. AIDS is bringing us full circle. Today there is much greater knowledge and skill in the realm of physical healing, but in many cases that is not enough: We are having to reawaken to the other aspects of balancing that allow our PWAs health in spite of their illness.

For example, the healing potency of simple physical touch has been awe-inspiring to those of us who work in the field. Sometimes, when no words could work, an understanding touch to a PWA's hand seemed to relieve the dis-ease. On another level, healing for some PWAs and their families is a joint process of learning to feel together—pain, grief, laughter, frustration, and whatever else comes along, to fully feel and share the experiences without judging the feelings as weak or wrong.

Our experience has been that true healing often begins at the moment the PWA decides to take full *responsibility* (not blame) for the disease and for his/her health. The healing for the family, we find, begins when they decide to take full *responsibility* for the fact that though the disease is happening to the PWA, everybody is affected and therefore involved with the healing process, regardless of where it ends. Taking responsibility is not the same as accepting (or laying on) blame or guilt; rather, it is acknowledging and participating in the *now,* in the well-being of the now, wherever that is to be found. Taking responsibility is making a conscious step out of the Drama Triangle, refusing to stay stuck as a Victim, Persecutor, or Rescuer. AIDS has no Victims when no one allows himself to be controlled by victim consciousness.

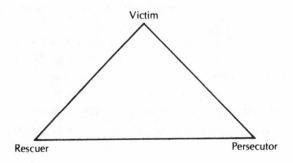

Healing is a challenging procedure when looked upon in its broad scope. It requires the full courage and determination of the PWA and family to learn to live each day to its fullest. It requires the PWA and family to love each other openly and honestly and nonjudgmentally, even in the times of despair and pain.

▪ THE PWA'S ▪
EXPERIENCE

At the point of being diagnosed, the PWAs are not only faced with a threat to their survival but also with changes in their health, lifestyle, social life, and goals for the future. In short, there is no aspect of a PWA's life that is not subject to total havoc; and what is not disrupted is always subject to the fear that it may yet be. They have reason for their fears. The disease can cause extreme physical pain, dementia, and loss of bodily functions. The disease causes loss of jobs and, consequently, medical coverage, life insurance protection, nonvested pension and profit-sharing benefits, and disability income; which leads to loss of savings, homes, cars, and possessions; which can lead to personal bankruptcy and welfare lines; which often causes loss of self-esteem, loss of friends, and sometimes even suicide.

Because AIDS is an epidemic disease, there is a great deal of public fear surrounding it, which leads to discrimination in housing, jobs, and even medical treatment. Because the disease was originally thought to be limited to homosexual men, IV-drug users, Haitians, and prostitutes, a social stigma has arisen that surrounds this disease unlike any other. This is the psychosocial nightmare of AIDS.

How an individual responds to the diagnosis and the fears it presents is predetermined by the personality of the individual. People use the coping skills they have learned to use previously during other challenges in their lives. For instance, those who have been independent will usually strive for their independence, while the person who has been dependent in life will expect others to supply care and make decisions. Those who have made close and intimate ties with family and friends will probably maintain those relationships, while those who have unsteady relationships may find support being withdrawn.

▪ STAGES OF EMOTIONAL RESPONSE ▪

Due to the "terminal" prognosis associated with AIDS, diagnosis can be catastrophic to the individual. At this point, to be protected emotionally, the PWA may respond through shock or disbelief. Many individuals may expect the bad news because they may not have felt well for quite some time; but the diagnosis confirms their worst fears, and shock and disbelief are still normal reactions.

The amount of stress the PWA feels at this time is directly related to the kind of support available from family and friends. People who are alone and isolated may become overwhelmed and immobilized.

After the initial shock and disbelief may come denial, an attempt to ignore or forget the diagnosis. Hiding in denial allows a person time to regroup and become prepared to deal with the challenges ahead. This is an especially difficult stage for the person with AIDS to maintain due to the widespread publicity and knowledge of the disease and the possibility of knowing friends and acquaintances with the disease. Rather than being able to hide and forget the reality for a while, the PWA may be forced to see it in his friends and on television.

After denial, a bargaining stage often occurs, hopefully followed with an ongoing commitment to work on the challenges at hand and toward recovery. Some PWAs, though, give up the struggle and never allow themselves to see beyond the possibility of their own demise.

The person with AIDS or ARC will likely respond to the experience with a wide range of emotions: anger, depression, fear, guilt, despair, anxiety, hurt, sadness; and at times, joy, peace, and happiness. These feelings change frequently and, if they become too intense, they can become immobilizing. Or, because it is possible to experience a combination of hopeful highs and hopeless lows at the same time, the PWA can become snared in the emotional confusion and be unable to move ahead with life.

▪ OTHER EMOTIONAL RESPONSES ▪

The majority of people diagnosed are young, previously healthy, and in the prime of life. It is a group whose thoughts are on their personal goals and aspirations rather than on the issues of mortality. They are faced with catastrophic changes in their personal and job relationships, in their physical bodies, and their self-images. Then, all of a sudden, they can experience a seemingly total loss of control in their lives. At the minimum, daily routine is disrupted; the unlucky lose their jobs. As income is disrupted or diminished, the PWA faces losing his or her personal possessions, everything the person may have concentrated on obtaining in life up to this point. With these losses generally comes social embarrassment and the lessening of self-esteem. The PWA in this situation often begins to feel either gypped by life or, conversely, totally deserving of the disease—in either case, victimized. In the worst cases, this leads to a complete social and/or geographic isolation.

For gay men, there may be a reliving of the "coming out" process, the process of accepting one's homosexuality. At diagnosis, many gay men reexamine their sexual identity. By associating AIDS with what society considers illicit, the PWA is faced with working through his guilt feelings again so that his sexual identity may be reaffirmed in such a way as to allow him to feel good about himself and his life.

Additionally, on receiving an AIDS diagnosis, many gay men are faced with disclosing their homosexuality to family, friends, and colleagues. If the PWA loses support due to these disclosures, his sense of guilt and victimization are verified externally and reinforced internally. Without a speedy resolution to all of these negative feelings, the PWA can sink into a morass of self-abasement and cease the struggle for his health. Too, in this black period is when some PWAs will look to suicide for relief.

PWAs are confronted with other people seeing them as "contagious," which will cause them to feel undesirable. This is another emotion that can cause a PWA to become isolated— emotionally, geographically, or both.

• ISOLATION •

One of the biggest and most destructive stressors faced is that of being isolated. At diagnosis, people with AIDS or ARC have an increased need for physical contact and emotional intimacy. But during this time, out of fear and a sense of helplessness, lovers, family, and friends may withdraw their support.

There are few PWAs who have been fortunate enough to have never lost someone close to them at this juncture. When this happens, the PWA is, of course, going to feel alone and isolated. This feeling may be enhanced by any emotions that arose in the normal processes previously described. In this case, the PWA may feel the need (real or imagined) to create new means of support at a time when there may not be the physical energy available to do so. Feeling the need and not being able to do anything about it simply amplifies the sense of aloneness.

If the PWA is required to be hospitalized, the isolation from friends and daily routine can become intensified. In situations where hospital personnel and visitors are required to wear gowns, masks, and gloves, the sense of isolation can become complete and even dehumanizing.

Outside the hospital, the general public has not responded to AIDS patients as it has to others who are ill, and at times, services (police, ambulance, medical, and even burial) have been withheld. PWAs are often denied benefits, employment, and care, a situation that is especially true for PWARCs, whose AIDS-related conditions do not have even the few legal protections allowed full-blown AIDS patients.

The sexual and personal precautions the PWAs must take to protect themselves and others certainly underscore the feelings of being "different" and alone. For many, there may be a complete change of sexual attitude, patterns, and habits: an entirely new way of relating to others. As old patterns may be unsafe and new patterns untried and clumsy, there may be a great deal of fear or difficulty in becoming sexual or intimate. If the PWA associates the disease with his/her previous sexual behavior, the difficulties may be magnified through guilt. Even some of those in monogamous relationships may face these problems: whether to have sex, what is safe, and how to deal with each other's anxieties. Sometimes, the stress can seem so overwhelming that attempting activity together just does not seem worth it.

▪ FEELING DEPENDENT ▪

In addition to having to rely more heavily on family and friends for emotional support, many people with AIDS are faced with applying for social services for the first time. Many of the PWAs have been economically independent and even well-to-do. Many come from families who looked down upon those who did have to seek these services as being people unwilling to work. The experience of applying for social services is almost always frustrating and demoralizing.

In many areas, one is required to be at the welfare office by 8:00 A.M. in order to make application, but then be required to wait until 3:30 P.M. to see anyone. They then may be treated like just another number in an overburdened system, being told that certain forms are not complete (which may mean doing the process again after a week's delay), and being informed that there is no assistance available (especially for PWARCs). If welfare is available, there is often a delay of six weeks before it begins.

Additionally, there is the conflict between continuing to work and remaining self-sufficient or forgoing work in order to be eligible for services. The public systems generally leave few halfway measures that allow for a decreasing work schedule.

Applying for help is one thing; accepting and using the services is another. The first time a formerly independent person uses food stamps at his local store or cashes a welfare check at his local bank is often traumatic. It may be viewed by the PWA as a public admission of illness and an acceptance of the role of a "charity case."

There is a final aspect of dependence that is the most frustrating of all: the fear of a protracted illness that will drain family and friends financially as well as emotionally. This frustration is widely recognized as a major cause of suicide among seriously ill people.

■ THE POSITIVE EXPERIENCE ■

The PWA's experience need not be as gloomy as it might seem from reading these pages. The PWA will face problems due to the disease; but with help from family and friends, what could be tragedies are frequently turned around into positive challenges. Many PWAs gain a sense of personal strength by going through these waters: Many never realized the strength they command. Others learn for the first time how to accept assistance and love from people who care, a lesson that makes life so much more pleasant and fulfilling when learned. Support can come from the most unlikely places, and that, too, is a learning experience.

One of the family's—whether it be the biological family or a support structure of loved ones or a fusion of both—primary functions is to support the PWA in finding solutions. That is accomplished through lending encouragement, being loving, remaining positive, and finding the humor in snarled situations. For some reason, when the PWA reaches a point where grim situations yield laughter rather than anger, doors just seem to open and support pops up. When the family is supportive and caring, it becomes really difficult for the PWA to become mired in the darkness for very long.

▪ THE FAMILY'S ▪
EXPERIENCE

The family, whatever that entity happens to be, will be where the PWA will turn for help and guidance; it may also be the place where the PWA vents his or her own grief, anger, frustration, and guilt. To handle the reality of the PWA's physical illness and emotional reactions, and to deal with your own emotional crises, all while trying to maintain a stable life may seem overwhelming.

In the section above, the PWAs' experiences were explained so that you would know what they are experiencing in order that you be better able to deal with them and to enable you to recognize what lies behind an angry word or an expression of desperation. Many of those feelings are obvious when they are set forth: it's obvious that a person with a terminal diagnosis is going to feel anger and that people who are trying to help him or her may get a dose of it!

Less obvious are the reactions that you will experience by placing yourself in the caregiving role, the psychological and social challenges that you as a family member will face during the illness and thereafter. But, knowing what these are allows you to keep them in perspective when they happen and keeps them from taking control and immobilizing you. As a member of the caregiving family, your well-being is critical to the PWA's health.

▪ DEFINING THE FAMILY ▪

The family that is asked to go through the healing process with the PWA may be any group of people who think of the PWA as a loved one. It may be family of origin: mother, father, and siblings. It may include extended family: aunts, uncles, grandparents, cousins, and so on. Or it may be comprised partially or solely of unrelated members of a current household (e.g., roommate), a significant other—whether living in the household or not (e.g., lover, best friend, etc.)—or people brought together by the illness (e.g., nurses, volunteer caregivers, etc.).

The term "family" as used here includes all those people who decide to go through this experience *with* their loved one. It is a *unit* that professionals agree has a great deal of influence in creating an atmosphere conducive to healing in its truest sense. This family is presently the strongest medicine available to us in the fight against AIDS!

As the family is a unit working together with a common goal, it is important that you work together, supporting and nurturing each member. Often people of diverse backgrounds are together in the family, and this may be present some difficulties. For instance, parents may be required to work closely with their child's lover. We have observed that, because of the common bond shared in everyone's love for the PWA, all *can* work together.

▪ EMOTIONAL RESPONSES ▪

The shock and disbelief you can experience when first hearing a loved one has AIDS or ARC is often accompanied by a sense of helplessness and fear, even panic. The reality that AIDS brings into the family taps your deepest feelings, fears, and unresolved questions about drug usage, homosexuality, infectious and life-threatening disease, death, religion, personal ethics—many of the value-laden issues of our lifetime.

Fear regarding the outcome of the illness is natural. The uncertainty of the unknown future can be terrifying. But in addition, there comes fear of the disease itself. Can I catch this disease? Will it spread to the children? These fears, too, are natural.

After the initial shock wears off, a variety of emotions may arise: intense hurt, embarrassment, anger, and/or guilt. Betty-Clare Moffatt writes in *When Someone You Love Has AIDS,* "I was in shock. I walked around for days, angry, angry, angry. . . ." These feelings can seem overwhelming and out of place, interfering with your desire to remain constructive. But, understand that these, too, are natural and human feelings that accompany change and loss.

Specifically, there may be a loss or change of an image that had been held of a son or daughter prior to the illness that the reality of AIDS alters. For instance, the family may learn that their PWA had been seriously involved with IV-drug usage, which may have resulted in the AIDS diagnosis. When the image of the wholesome child is marred, there will generally be an emotional response. These emotions are a natural part of grieving.

The emotions discussed so far have been spurred by the diagnosis, a reaction to the disease. There is another set of emotions that arises due to the stigma of the disease and to societal pressures. If the PWA is a relative or if the PWA is living with you, your entire social life may change drastically. Besides the direct responsibilities of dealing with an ill person, there is often the embarrassment factor for the family of the PWA. Because people are afraid of AIDS, you may not feel comfortable telling your friends and neighbors why they can't drop over anymore, or how you are spending your evenings. You may resort to "white lies" about your son or daughter having "cancer," and you may begin to dislike yourself for the stories you feel compelled to tell. This, too, is human and very common. Its real danger is that it leads to the very isolation and social ostracism (though self-induced) that the stories were designed to protect against!

Without neighbors and friends who know the circumstances, there may be no place for you to turn for comfort, assistance, and support. Without those outlets, the stresses you are likely to feel due to your loved one having the disease will simply increase more rapidly and lead to burnout. The cases of neighbors turning their backs are far outnumbered by the stories of neighbors and friends showing in countless ways their true depth of caring and support for families of AIDS patients. Besides, if you can't count on your friends in a crisis (and this is a crisis!), why would you want to play bridge with them?

On the other side of the coin, many members of the family

feel that AIDS was visited on their loved one due to that person's lifestyle—be that sexual promiscuity, homosexual activity, or IV-drug usage. It may be that you do not approve of that lifestyle and want to "protect" your PWA from any more "contamination" from "those people." Too often, a PWA loses his or her natural support systems because family members close the doors to the PWA's friends. Blaming others, anyone, for the disease will not assist in healing it. Indeed, your ostracism will cause everyone's stress levels to increase and actually helps promote the disease. The PWA needs the support systems that have been part of his/her life before; and the family needs them, too! Throughout all of this, the family members will question their economic resources, their ability to work with a terminally ill person and still earn a living, and eventually, the whole point of life. There are no easy answers to these questions, though some of the other chapters in this book point toward solutions. Know, though, that this type of questioning, and finding our *own* answers, is not only natural and normal, but part of what growth is about for each of us.

▪ GUIDANCE FOR THE FAMILY ▪

To this point, this chapter has dealt with what the PWA and his or her family (regardless of who those people are) may feel and what they may experience. The purpose has not been neither to scare anyone nor to suggest that everyone will experience the same things. Rather, the point has been to acquaint you with them so that, if they do crop up in your experience, you will not feel alone or insane. By recognizing what is happening within you, it becomes easier to work with the experience or feeling to resolve it quickly and comfortably.

What follows from this point is a list of pointers that may ease you through this crisis with your PWA. Many of these are developed more fully in other chapters, and many need only be mentioned to bring them into consciousness and use.

▪ MAINTAINING OPEN COMMUNICATIONS ▪

Communications are easily snarled in any crisis situation. We get rushed and forget, or we tell only a part of the situation and expect others to fill in the gaps, or we hedge and tell less than the whole truth in order to spare ourselves or others. Bad communications lead to troubles and emotional garbage. Emotional garbage leads to stress and health problems. It is mandatory to be open, forthright, and honest at all levels, beginning with yourself.

Since public misinformation is common, your friends and neighbors will look to you for correct information concerning AIDS. Indeed, you may have to provide information for your PWA as well. It is important for you to stay abreast of the most current knowledge and communicate what you learn. This will not only allay your own fears but it will also make life easier on the families who come after you.

With regard to friends, neighbors, and other members of the family unit, let them know what they can do to help and what you expect of them. The people who offer to help really want to help: They're not just being polite. Let them. Allowing them to help when they want gives them a chance to feel good about contributing and allows the pressure on you and the other primary caregivers to be lessened. Along this line, ask for help when you need it. Many people that you would have expected to offer their help may have held back for fear of "intruding." Asking is not always easy, but the risk is almost always rewarding. Also, it is part of honest communicating.

Continue open communications by giving people concrete ways to assist when they ask (or you ask them); it decreases confusion. For instance, have them help with grocery shopping, household duties, spending special times with the PWA, preparing and delivering meals, and so on. If you hope that they will second-guess your needs, you may end up with a houseful of flowers but a sinkful of dishes.

Maintaining open communications with medical personnel

is a multifaceted project. First, it means coming up with a family plan in which the PWA is the central force. Then, it means communicating that plan to everyone involved so that there is no confusion of which treatments are going to be followed and how care is going to be administered. Often, this means that you will have to be an advocate for the PWA. Confronting the confusion and depersonalization inherent in the medical industry is difficult for most healthy people; it can be impossible for the PWA and his closest caregivers. Therefore, the burden may need to fall on others: Find a willing volunteer and let them see to it.

Often PWAs are unable to really understand what information they are receiving from their physicians. Part of the patient advocacy process is to have a person take notes and ask questions to relay to the rest of the family. Generally, the medical professionals will appreciate it, for part of the difficulty (and liability) they face is due to improper communications.

Remember that most people are really interested in providing proper care. Maintaining good relationships with the medical personnel (doctors, nurses, aides, even janitors) will help in fulfilling the needs and *rights* of your PWA.

Maybe the most challenging task will be to maintain honest communications with the PWA you love. Most of us want to believe that our loved ones will live forever. The reality of dealing with a life-threatening disease opens us to thoughts and feelings about our great taboo: death. Seeing the potential loss so close to us brings these feelings to the surface. Trying to keep these feelings bottled up is not healthy for you or those with whom you are in contact. Dishonesty about the *possibility* of another infection or death will only distance your relationship from the PWA.

It often feels "safest" to back off and avoid communicating with the PWA, especially if the person is newly diagnosed and riding the emotional roller coaster of hope and despair. To broach some subjects may be frighteningly painful, draining, and confusing to watch. Remember, though, that you are not the cause of the mood swings, that they are part of the disease. Actually, your being there helps the PWA to move through his or her feelings rather than keeping them bottled up for fear of hurting you! Often, just being able to *say* a feeling out loud helps to decrease its intensity.

On a practical level, communicating with the PWA helps make daily life easier. For instance, exploring both your needs together and the options for meeting them is healthy for you both. Practical issues may be those relating to visitation, financial matters, and decisions about life support, as well as what to eat and how to cook it. Often, it is not practical for you to meet everything that is desired or wanted by your PWA, and saying so allows care to continue without sacrifice or martyrdom.

There are times, however, when communicating means being quiet. It often means listening and hearing what is being said beneath the actual words. It will certainly mean *not* communicating judgments about the PWA's lifestyle, which you may feel led to the disease: That is the surest way to close communications. Instead, the time you have together can be better used in recognizing the connections and love you share, which are so much more important than any disagreements you may have. With thoughts and feelings verbalized respectfully, other considerations fall into their proper perspective.

Communicating openly and honestly may be a new experience for all concerned:

> "I took him in my arms and we both cried, the first time we had held each other and the first time we had cried together since he was a little boy." (Moffatt)

Touching and crying and laughing together are true forms of communicating. They are honest and pure and often say more than the spoken word. These forms of communication may be especially difficult for adult men; but it has been our experience that their touch, tears, and laughter are particularly valued by the PWA.

▪ MAINTAINING SUPPORT ▪

Much of maintaining support is intertwined with what was said previously about communicating. But, in addition to that, it will be necessary to work with the PWA and the other family members to make certain that support systems for everyone have not fallen through.

Regarding the PWA, part of the supportive role of the family involves reinforcing participation in the PWA's chosen therapies. These may include treatments, certain medications or diets, or alternative therapies like massage, acupuncture, healing visualizations, affirmations, and so on. Reinforcement means maintaining a positive outlook about the present treatments while being willing to explore new avenues. It means having consideration for the needs related to the therapies, such as a quiet time, making doctor's appointments, and so on. And sometimes it means making certain that the treatments are continued regularly: PWAs often want to give up before a treatment has a chance to do its work. Reinforcement means making certain your PWA gets exercise and eats to the best of his or her ability. It means helping him or her maintain dignity by not "babying," and encouraging the strength to refuse the "victim" role. And very often, it means finding ways to create laughter to ease the seriousness of the situation.

Supporting yourself is of primary concern: It is a combination of rest, exercise, taking time for yourself away from the PWA and the rest of the family. It means using outside support groups, either professionals or friends, to help you deal with the questions that death and disease bring to the top. It means reviewing spiritual matters within yourself as well as practical ones.

As regards the other caregivers, all of you will need to make certain that each is being supported individually so that there are no weak links in the system. In addition to that, the family itself will need to divide up the support management that will be required to make certain that legal matters are in order, financial concerns are met, housing and in-bed care planned, resources located, and required forms filled out and processed, all while normal daily activities and fun outings are continued. This requires time management on everyone's part. Support involves creative problem solving, open sharing, and remembering that everyone's needs have to be met. The key is forming and utilizing a broad base of support to reduce the stress for any single individual or group.

▪ WHAT IT ALL ▪ MEANS

Illness and death have been called the great teachers, though the lessons to be learned are different for everyone. Those of us working in the field have seen PWAs find their meaning in simply being able to *belong,* in groups or in their own families, grieving and receiving support. It may have been something these people had never had but found through their illness. We have seen PWAs who learned that the meaning they were seeking had to do with learning to fight, to stand up for themselves and gain a form of self-esteem they had never experienced.

Many have found that a new purpose for them was learning that they and others (including mom and dad) were human and made mistakes: Many learned to forgive and to experience *unconditional love.*

For some PWAs and family, the lesson is to learn to let go: to let go of controlling or, possibly, to let go of a life—their own or another's. It is a matter of realizing that no one really has any control over who is saved and who is not; that guilt accomplishes nothing, while love accomplishes miracles.

There is healing available for all of us who go through the AIDS process. It is found in experiencing the true meaning of one's personal power: to love even through despair and to trust in a Higher Power, or the Life Process itself, when everything else seems to be stripped away. It is the power obtained in all the new beginnings that are continually created in the *now.* It is the power to know that we can create good for ourselves in spite of what we encounter.

Though most of the suggestions in this chapter are practical and concrete, it is our hope that the *spirit* of the message comes through above it all. Regardless of what is faced by the PWA and family, regardless of what modern medicine is unable to cure, we know that the disease can be healed: we have seen it happen over and over again. It is what keeps us working in the field. It's more than a hope; it's a reality.

▪ BIBLIOGRAPHY ▪

Forstein, Marshall, M.D. "Psychosocial Impact of the Acquired Immunodeficiency Syndrome." *Seminars in Oncology,* March 1984, vol. II, no. 1, pp. 77–83.

Gong. *Understanding AIDS.* *

Hay. *You Can Heal Your Life.* *

Moffatt. *When Someone You Love Has AIDS.* *

———, ed. *AIDS: A Self Care Manual.* * (Previously: AIDS Project of Los Angeles. *Living with AIDS: A Self Care Manual.* This edition is out of print.)

Nichols, Stuart E., M.D. "Psychosocial Reactions of Persons with Acquired Immunodeficiency Syndrome." *Annals of Internal Medicine,* American Conference of Physicians. 1985, 103: 765–767.

Ryan. *Wellness Workbook.* *

Segal. *A Personal Program to Speed Healing and Enhance Wellness.* *

Simonton, C. *Getting Well Again.* *

Simonton, S. *The Healing Family.* *

Wein, Ken, Ph.D. and Diego Lopez, CSW. "Overview of Psychosocial Issues Concerning AIDS." *Psychiatric Annals,* March 1986, vol. 16, no. 3.

(Full bibliographical information may be found in Appendix F.)

6

· STORIES FROM · THE FRONT: NUMBER 1 DANIEL, MY SON

AMELIA LONDON

Amelia London resides alone in Dallas. During Daniel's illness, she became involved with establishing a Parents of PWAs Support Group, a project that continues to consume much of her time.

Daniel had been in the hospital for several days before the doctor's report was prepared. One night, when I went home, it was there waiting for me:

"Prognosis: TERMINAL"

I read that word—saw it in print. It was the most devastating moment of my life. The tears came. I screamed. I cried. I prayed. I was in pain and I was alone. Waves of nausea came over me. Sleep did not come until much, much later.

I would have gladly exchanged my life for his, but that was not to be. My son was dying. Every emotion known came through me. I was angry and frightened, feeling guilty and trapped and betrayed. I have heard that some parents directed these feelings toward their son. That I don't understand: My love for Daniel was the one constant emotion I could rely on at that time. I did not stop loving my son; I drew closer to him.

While he was still in the hospital, he asked his two brothers and me to come in to have the doctor talk to us about this disease: We knew so little about AIDS. It was heartbreaking for all of us, but his brothers were extremely supportive as were their wives and grown children. Rather than causing the family to run, the disease caused us to love Daniel and each other even more.

On his return home, we worked together on his diet and general health care. We had received instructions from the hospital before Daniel was discharged, as well as information about the various agencies we could tap, social workers, legal matters, and so on.

So my son came home to the room he had had since he was six years old, here to live for the short time he had left in this life. I thanked God each day that I was able to care for him, for in this time we got reacquainted. I got to know Daniel as an adult and not the little boy that I sent off to school every morning. That is not to say that there were not rough spots: Each of us had a period of adjusting. Daniel had been living independently in another city for several years: Being dependent on Mom, again, wasn't easy for him. In the meantime, I had been living alone in my own home and had become independent as well: Living with my son again wasn't easy for me! We cooperated with each other in every respect as far as his illness was concerned. However, we would have a little spat every now and then and pout around for an hour or so; then things would start flowing in the normal manner. I think we were normal in this.

When he came home from the hospital, he was frail and weak, but as time passed he grew stronger and gained weight. In fact, he looked better than he had in years! It was easy to forget that he had AIDS; it was a relief to have hope.

The first week we were home was topsy-turvy. Someone

called from some agency and made an appointment to call on us a few days later. On the day they were to come, we were waiting and Daniel said, "Who is this organization coming out?" I told him I didn't know and that I couldn't even remember the people's names. But, we both agreed that—Who cares?—we needed help and information: We were willing to reach out to anyone or anybody. As it turned out, it was the Visitation Committee of the AIDS Resource Center. This was the first encounter we had with any organized group, and we came to love those generous people.

They helped us in so many ways: financially for a short time and with food every so often. Most importantly, it was the people themselves who were so helpful, taking Daniel out, when he was able, to picnics, theater, and so on, and even spraying the yard for fleas once (Daniel came home with his pup).

Later the Oak Lawn Counseling Center took over and assigned two permanent "buddies" through their AIDS Project: Dru and Carla. I cannot even begin to tell what their loving care came to mean to Daniel and me. They were more than friends; they became a type of extended family.

Daniel was an expert when it came to maintenance here in my home. As it turned out, Dru was quite capable in this area, too. So it wasn't unusual to see the two of them working on some project together: up in the attic working on the air ducts, on the roof patching a leak that had developed next to the vent, many things too numerous to mention. As Daniel became weaker, Dru did more of the work with Daniel supervising. Even when Daniel became too weak to even do that, he had written notes and Dru carried on alone!

Carla, meanwhile, did many things for us. I remember one day she came over, giving me a chance to simply go to the grocery store. When I returned, there was Carla, washing the dishes. She would pick up Daniel's medications from the pharmacy, cook his favorite dishes, fold the laundry—so many things. All of this meant so much to me, for there were times at the end of the day that I was so emotionally and physically exhausted that all I could do was fall into bed.

They both pitched in wherever they could, as long-time friends would do. Dru did so much fixing up around the house because, like Daniel, he enjoyed it and because he realized that Daniel was trying to get things in order for me. So on a very real basis, these two became family.

It was not all work when they were here. There were happy times and laughter with an uplifting feeling for us during these very traumatic days. When Daniel felt like it, they took him out to movies, dinner, support groups, whatever. Carla took Daniel to a Halloween party just nine days before he died. The photographs of the party—seeing Daniel laughing and enjoying himself—are a continuing spirit-lifter for me.

The Oak Lawn Counseling Center was also important to us due to their AIDS support groups, for both PWAs and family. It was the first place I knew to go where people understood AIDS and weren't afraid of it. My first meeting there for "Friends and Relatives of PWAs" was informative and, at times, even comical. At one point, the subject got around to the kinds of care they were giving their PWA friends or relatives, and some of them started talking about how they had slipped into the habit of waiting on their PWA. It's a normal thing for us to do for our loved one, I thought, though I can understand why is it not in either's best interest.

When they got around to me and asked me what I was doing, I said, "Yes, I wait on him." The chairperson asked what kinds of things I did. I was so caught off guard that I couldn't think of the things I really was doing. So, I said, "I take his coffee into him every morning." Then the chairperson asked whether I had Daniel do anything for me. "Oh, yes," I replied; but by now my mind had stopped. "Like what?" he asked. "Well, I went to bed one night and my TV remote control was on the dresser and I asked Daniel to hand it to me as he went to his room." The group got a chuckle out of that, and I realized that everyone in that room understood what I was saying (or not saying) because they had all been where I was.

When Daniel grew stronger, he did maintenance around the house, as I said: all of the things I couldn't remember to tell the

Friends and Relatives group that night. Also, he began volunteering in the AIDS Clinic at Parkland Hospital and devoted several hundred hours there that year. He became familiar with the progress of the other patients, so he knew what was happening to his own body as his disease progressed.

As the months passed, Daniel grew weaker. He spent more time at home and we had more time together. Though there were stretches of grief and pain, I do not think of our time together as negative. My son had a unique sense of humor and a way of expressing himself that rubbed off on all of us, even his dog, who keeps my spirits up today with her comedy. We laughed a lot over small things.

I remember one day when I was ready to change the linens and took the sheets into his room to ask whether he wanted these sheets with large butterflies on them. He said yes; then I asked him which way he wanted the butterflies to fly: toward him or away from him. He replied that he would prefer them toward him. This was all a very serious question-and-answer session; and then we both heard how ridiculous we must have sounded and laughed until our sides ached.

Then one day, he was hurting so very much. And he looked up and said, "I'll tell you one thing: I'll never go through this again." He thought about what he had said, and then added wryly, "Guess I'll never have the chance."

We had much time to talk; we grew close as mother and son and confidant. He became more spiritual as time went by. He openly talked of this and I was glad. I did not press my beliefs on him for fear that it would hold him back or make him think that I was making some sort of judgment. I loved him too much to judge and, oh God, he was dying!

One of my favorite things to remember—and I always get a smile on my face—was one morning when he was sitting at the breakfast table quietly, he looked up suddenly and said, "I'll tell you one thing. I've been reading that Bible over there. Revelations. And it follows this AIDS thing. And, frankly, we only have about three pages to go!" Later in the day, I thought about what he had said and it came to mind that the Bible he had been reading was my Bible with the extra-large print; and maybe we didn't have but one more page to go in regular print! I didn't tell him this because he had been so serious.

There are times in the middle of the pain when the only thing to do is laugh. Sometimes it seems like black humor; but it was a choice of laughing or crying, and I cried enough as it was. Toward the very end, when his health started to deteriorate rapidly, Daniel was unable to lift himself from the bed. He had always taken care of his own medication, but he was also becoming forgetful. I asked him whether he would like me to count it out for him. Daniel half-lifted one hand and pointed a weak, shaky finger at me and said, "Don't you start treating *me* like an *invalid!*"

He had great pride and was concerned about losing his faculties. My heart went out to him. About this time, he could hardly swallow his food: Sometimes it took two hours to eat a meal. How I suffered for him and with him! He had tried AZT, but his body and system could not handle it. From then on, it was all downhill. He began to lose more weight, grow weaker, and become more disoriented. One morning, about two-thirty, I was awakened by the front door being opened, and at the same moment, he cried, "Mom!" I jumped out of bed and ran to the living room, where he was standing in the middle of the floor. Both the patio door and front door were wide open. I said, "What happened, honey?" He said he had been looking for me. When I told him I was in bed, he said that he had looked in my room and that I was not there!

He had only his shorts on and he was ice-cold, having a chill. He had evidently looked for me outdoors; I do not know for how long or where he went. I got him back to bed and turned the electric blanket on until the chill finally subsided and he went to sleep. The next day, Daniel did not remember anything about the previous night.

I wasn't ready for this kind of thing to happen and it was heartrending for me. But, all through the illness the most unexpected things happened. At the beginning, a young woman had been sent out by one of the agencies on a temporary assignment.

She was wonderful and she and Daniel grew to like each other a lot. Even after her assignment was over, she came by daily. But at some point, it got out of hand: She fell in love with Daniel, knowing that he was dying and knowing his lifestyle! That created a lot of problems that no one knew how to handle.

Also unexpected was the fact that Daniel's two closest, life-long friends absolutely deserted him when they learned he had AIDS. Daniel was crushed and there was nothing I could do. Whether it was their fear of getting the disease or some other reason, I don't know. But the pain it caused was almost unforgivable. If there is one lesson you learn from reading this, let it be here: Don't desert the people who love you when they need you!

There were times when he was in the very depths of despair, especially at night. He would play very soft music and listen for hours with his lights dimmed. He would sit with his knees up and with his head resting on his arms, almost in a fetal position. When I went in and saw him, I would quietly walk out. This was a time of prayer and meditation for him, but it was a heartbreaking picture for me.

The stress and heartbreak added up and tears would come at any moment, day or night, in the car, in the store, while doing housework, just anytime. I coped to the best of my ability, for at that time there was not much support for a parent. The Friends and Relatives group still met weekly, but it was mostly men: I needed to talk with another mother! But while Daniel was volunteering in the AIDS Clinic, he met the mother of one of the patients. He gave her my phone number and she contacted me. We later met—each of us with our PWA sons—had a lovely lunch, and made arrangements to keep in contact. We did maintain the contact throughout the deaths of both of our sons (her son died twenty-six days before Daniel did), and from that has grown a small group of parents who meet on a regular basis.

Three of the sons of parents in our group have already died. Each of the parents has his or her own way of handling the grief before and after death. We talk it out and give comfort to one another, and it helps a great deal. It doesn't matter that we are a group of such different people, professionally, religiously, and economically; we are a group of people with a common bond: our PWAs, our sons.

My last conversation with Daniel is a memory I will treasure forever. He was in pain, he was hurting, but he wanted to talk. I sat in the chair beside his bed. We talked about many things. He wanted me to know how much he appreciated and thanked me for caring for him. His one great concern was how I was going to make it after he was gone. I tried to let him know that caring for him at this time was a privilege for me, that I would not have it any other way. I tried to tell him that my life would change and have new meaning for me—and it has! He gave me so much.

It seems as if we covered every facet of his life that night. It was like a spiritual awakening for me. There was a closeness of some kind that I never had in my life. Later, he said, "Why don't you sit on the foot of the bed?" I did, and leaned against the wall: We talked until 3 A.M. Then he said, "Mother, I want to pray." He went down to the end of the bed where I was sitting and laid his head on my shoulder; and I held him in my arms. He prayed to his Heavenly Father the most beautiful prayer I ever heard in my entire life. And, he ended the prayer with these words, "Mother, I'll be waiting for you." I think now, My God, what more could a parent ask of their dying child?

After the prayer he said, "You need some rest now," so I tucked him into his bed. He was propped up on two or three pillows and one arm was out of the covers. He was comfortable when I went to my room. I awakened three hours later at 6 A.M. and went in to check on him. He was in the same position as when I had left him, but he was in a coma, never to talk to me again.

I called the next-door neighbor and my daughter-in-law, both of whom are nurses, and both came immediately to take charge. Two days later, Daniel's brother had just finished shaving him when he quietly and gently passed away. All of us were there: my other two sons, my daughters-in-law, and me. When my son died, a part of me went with him. What is left of me has been enriched by him.

I have been asked what I would tell other parents who find

themselves where I have been. I don't know. These pages tell some of how I have been able to get to today. But I would tell them one final thing: Never contemplate what might happen tomorrow. The same everlasting Father who cares for you and your child today and every day will either shield you from suffering, or He will give you unfailing strength to bear it. He gave it to me in Daniel's last words: "Mother, I'll be waiting for you." I know I still have work to do in my life. I do it gladly and lovingly, knowing what awaits me at the end of my path.

Through this part of it, three months after Daniel's death, my one consolation is that one sentence, "Mother, I'll be waiting for you."

7

▪ PEER COUNSELING ▪

CANDICE J. MARCUM, M.ED., L.P.C.

Candice J. Marcum, M.Ed., L.P.C., is a psychotherapist in private practice in Dallas. One of the original core of counselors who opened the Oak Lawn
Counseling Center, Candy has been involved with
counseling those who are acting as caregivers since
the need first arose.

The caregivers who deal with persons with AIDS (PWAs) and
AIDS-Related Complex (PWARCs) are often called upon to be
counselors for the ill person. Whether one is a friend, relative,
or never-before-seen volunteer makes no difference. At some
point every caregiver hears some of the PWA's concerns and
worries.

Most of the caregivers have never had any formal training
in counseling. A psychology course or two in college can be
helpful but is generally not sufficient to make one feel comfortable counseling a person who is confronted with all of the conflicts of a terminal illness, especially AIDS. The purpose of this
chapter, therefore, is to give one the *practical* tools and understanding to feel comfortable in the counseling mode to offer
comfort and assistance to your PWA.

All of us know "natural" counselors. They are the people

who seem to be comfortable with other people when they are talking. If one observes "natural helpers" from a distance, one sees that they seem to pay close attention to what is being said. They do not interrupt and they maintain eye contact. Interestingly enough, these interpersonal skills were probably learned by these "naturals." In order to learn these skills, however, a person must have a desire to help.

The characteristics of this type of helping individual are warmth, empathy, and honesty combined with a caring nature and a feeling of respect for others. If this defines you, read on. You will make a wonderful counselor, if you were not one already!

If, however, these are not your strong points, you may wish to stay away from the counseling aspects of working with PWAs: There is so much else that needs to be done in order to maintain and enhance their quality of life for any of us to waste time and energy in areas where we are weak. Everyone has strengths, and everyone's strengths can be put to good use in the AIDS arena. Look elsewhere in this book to see how your strengths can best be used. Possibly, you are a natural organizer and businessman: You may want to administer the organizational matters spoken of in the chapter entitled "Things That Fall Through the Cracks." Or, you may be a more physical, hands-on type of person, and want to use your talents by assisting physically: Read the chapters entitled "AIDS 301: Alternative Therapies" and "Home Care of a PWA."

Part of peer counseling is sorting out who is best at doing what for whom!

▪ THE HELPING ▪
PROCESS

The helping process typically has three stages to it. It may be looked at as exploring a problem, understanding a problem, and acting on a problem. Or, it may be seen as defining a problem, goal development for resolving a problem, and taking action toward that goal. At least, this is the way in which most of us look at resolving our own problems.

MODEL A:
EXPLORING   UNDERSTANDING   ACTING

MODEL B:

STAGE I: PROBLEM DEFINITION
STAGE II: GOAL DEVELOPMENT
STAGE III: ACTION

The counselor, however, looks at helping another person solve their problems, and has three slightly different stages to their problem solving:

MODEL C:
PROBLEM
ASSISTING
OUTCOME

For the counselor, the process begins when someone has a *problem* or concern; that is, a person believes that "Things are not as I want them to be." The "things" may be feelings, other people, financial conditions, or any multitude of factors. So, the first stage is still defining the problem to some degree; but it goes on to include understanding what that problem involves.

Assisting involves the counselor's use of helping tools, skills, and strategies directed toward the other person's concerns. Here, helping tools are generally pieces of information—how to get Social Security income, for example. It is the data bank. Helping skills are what this chapter is all about: The skills that a person uses, verbally or nonverbally, to help another person (the PWA or PWARC) clarify the problem in his/her own mind in order to come to an understanding of the problem and solutions. A strategy is a plan of action to be followed in solving or resolving the problem ideas (e.g., suggesting a way to resolve a parent-child conflict), and *skills* (e.g., clarifying a complex idea). A *strategy* is a plan for using the tools.

The helping process ends when a desired *outcome* has occurred and the person being helped can say, "Things have changed —they are more like I want them to be."

When in the role of counselor with a PWA, one of the most important things we can do is to understand the PWA's problem by seeing the world (and thus the problems) through his/her eyes. This means getting to know the problem, not only as it may sound to be but also as it may feel to be. We must see the world through the PWA's eyes before we can filter his/her experience of it through our own eyes.

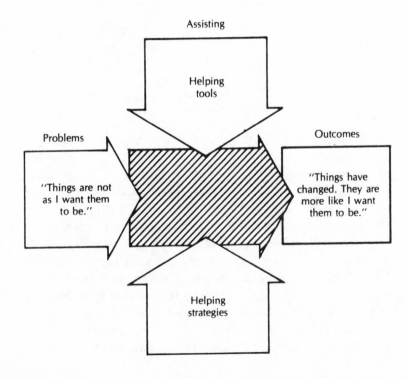

Assisting

Helping tools

Problems

"Things are not as I want them to be."

Outcomes

"Things have changed. They are more like I want them to be."

Helping strategies

All of us have had the "helpful friend" who understands our problem only too well . . . generally before we have explained it to them. And, they have this week's miracle answer on the tip of their tongue: "All you need is elixir of frog hair!" The PWA often feels that no one understands his or her problems and, therefore, may think of each of us as "helpful friends." To a great extent, s/he is right. This is why the counselor must make every effort to understand what the PWA *really* does feel. This means listening attentively, paying attention to the PWA in many ways. What people say and how they say it tells us a great deal about how they see themselves and the world around them. In addition to listening carefully, the counselor will also be required to observe the PWA on a number of levels in order to see how s/he *functions.* Does it really connect with what s/he says? Does it correspond to what s/he or you think s/he feels? What people say is interesting; what they do is truth.

▪ SKILLS OF A HELPER ▪

Most of what has been said before and what will come hereafter deals with material you already know. It discusses methods and skills that you likely use on a daily basis unwittingly and well. The purpose of putting it all down in black and white is not to teach you what you already know but, in a sense, to remind you of what you know.

When you are dealing with a PWA who is terminally ill or a PWARC who is worried that s/he may be terminally ill, the kind of problems that surface are much more weighty than the problems we are used to counseling. How a bedridden person is going to make ends meet seems to be a much graver problem than that of a healthy friend who has recently lost a job and is concerned about making ends meet. When called upon to counsel in situations of this gravity, we often feel unqualified. "These are life-and-death matters. What can I do? I'm a peer, not a professional!" This is both true and untrue. By reminding you of skills you already have, you will come to know that you are much more capable of helping than you may think.

Of course, you may feel unprepared and unknowledgeable about some of the PWA's problems. This is understandable and correct. There are people in your community who are better prepared and better educated to whom you can turn both for information and skills. Get to know the resources available in your area that deal with PWAs and their problems. This is where you will find your new helping tools. Acquaint yourself with the colleges, churches, and hospitals in your area. These facilities will have professionals on staff who can help you and guide you with your helping skills. Do not be shy in asking for help: That is what these people and agencies are for. Remember to keep a list of the names and phone numbers of contacts you make to use again when the need arises.

The other reason for putting down in black and white what you already know about counseling is to give you a place to go for answers when you become confused or stumped. The problems faced by the PWA or PWARC, as well as the family and friends, are legion. Often, what seems to be a small problem is the tip of the iceberg. Often, the counselor may be overwhelmed in simply trying to define the problem. That is when the peer counselor can turn back to these pages to see what skill or strategies or tools s/he can use effectively to simplify and clarify.

At this point we are going to shift focus. Heretofore, there has been an overt recognition of you—the counselor—as a peer (friend or associate) of a PWA or PWARC, as well as of his family and friends, most likely. This recognition presupposes a certain bonding between you and the PWA, so that his problems become yours emotionally. But to be an effective counselor requires a degree of objectivity. Objectivity, in turn, presupposes a certain amount of detachment.

From this point on, we are going to help you build that sense of detachment: It will be assumed that you are a professional counselor dealing with a paying client. More than seeking objectivity, we are after a shift in perspective.

The difference between the professional counselor and the peer counselor can be seen on a couple of levels. The professional counselor is required to live up to an objective and an externally enforced code of ethics. The peer counselor has personal ethics, no doubt; but personal ethics are not as impartial as externally enforced codes of ethics. Compare this with the differences between the artist and the artisan. An artist, no matter how good or bad, is allowed to create fully to his personal satisfaction. The artisan is required to perform and create to the satisfaction of his clients. Often the peer counselor's major difficulty will be in knowing who s/he is representing amongst all of his/her peers. Is the problem that is being worked on, for which a resolution is sought, that of the PWA, the family, friends, or yours?

Example. You have been with your PWA for several hours at the hospital. You are tired and want to go home. Your PWA wants you to stay because he is expecting a difficult encounter with a family member and wants you to be a referee. Additionally, the doctor has not yet made an appearance, and there is certain information that you feel you should know and that you are afraid you may be unable to obtain third-hand from your PWA later. Do you stay or do you go? If you stay, are you being "used" in your role as referee? Are there some items that need to be worked out between the PWA and the family member without your presence? Will the family require that the PWA remain in the hospital instead of going home if you are not there? Whose side are you on? Maybe you just want to leave because you are tired. Maybe it is best that you leave. The doctor may not come tonight, after all. Is this really a problem? Whose problem is it? Yours? The PWA's? The family's? The doctor's?

If you were, in fact, a professional counselor, you would most likely have established a strategy for the PWA (and for yourself, possibly) to follow in dealing with the family member. If you were, indeed, a professional counselor, you would probably not be awaiting the doctor's arrival, but, rather, would telephone the doctor for the information you seek.

Notice how placing yourself in a totally different perspective allows different solutions. That is the purpose in changing the focus.

There are five categories of counseling and problem-solving behavior to master. These are the abilities to:

1. listen actively to a client
2. reflect a client's verbal and nonverbal behavior
3. ask questions
4. summarize
5. help a client solve a problem

We will look at each of these separately.

SKILL 1. *Active listening* is designed to encourage the client to communicate more information. The more information the client shares, the easier it will be for the counselor to understand the client's problem. Active listening is also one way the counselor can show respect for the client. This can help prevent a feeling of mistrust on the part of the client toward the counselor. By preventing mistrust, active listening can lay the foundation for effective counselor-client relationships.

Active listening may be accomplished either verbally (e.g., "I see." "Um-hum.") or nonverbally (e.g., facial expression, posture).

SKILL 2. *Reflecting* is a method of editing and replaying to the client what you have seen in a client's nonverbal communication (e.g., "I notice when you mention your mom, you grin; when you mention your sister, you look away.") or heard in the client's verbal communication (e.g., "I hear a lot of pain in that anger."). Reflecting a client's verbal and nonverbal behavior is such an important counseling skill because it helps the client gain a clearer understanding of his/her behavior. It can also help the client become aware of the degree to which feelings mold his or her actions.

SKILL 3. *Questions.* Open-ended questions (e.g., "How do you feel about that?") are designed to help clients clarify their ideas and feelings. Closed-ended questions (e.g., "Who said that to you?"), in contrast, are designed to ask for factual information.

SKILL 4. *Summarizing* is an important helping skill because it provides an opportunity for the counselor to review with the client what has been said during the session and to tie it all together. Also, it allows both to remember what was said that led up to the summarization. For example, it is wise to summarize the alternatives that may be followed to resolve a problem and to ask the client to confirm or dispute your summary.

SKILL 5. *Problem Solving.* Many times a helper can teach a client how to problem-solve by following a systematic problem-solving process. In learning this process, the client may be better able to solve future problems without your assistance. One easy system is to use a "Problem-Solving Worksheet" like the one on page 118.

In completing a Problem-Solving Worksheet, the client will need to make a statement of the problem. The counselor will define the problem to his/her understanding and seek confirmation or denial from the client. With regards to the possible alternatives, write down every one that the client can think of, while remaining completely nonjudgmental. Only after all the alternatives are enumerated will the counselor begin to help the client in analyzing the possible consequences of each alternative. Ask the client what are the possible positive and negative effects of each alternative one-by-one and have him/her rate that alternative as excellent, fair, or poor.

When all the alternatives have been analyzed and rated, the

PROBLEM-SOLVING WORKSHEET

Client's Name: *John Doe*
Date: *Wed., May 5, 1988*
Helper: *Candy Marcum*

Problem: *Inability to sleep at night*

Alternatives	Excellent	Fair	Poor
#1. *Refuse to sleep during daytime*		X	
#2. *Talk to doctor*	X		
#3. *Exercise daily*		X	
#4. *Not worry about it*	X		
#5. *Take sleeping pills*			X

counselor asks the client to choose the best alternative(s) on the basis of the ratings. The client's decision needs to be supported by the counselor in order to instill confidence and to encourage the client to act on the decision reached.

There are two other skills that a professional counselor uses that are helpful to the peer counselor: starting and ending a session. Unlike the professional counselor, you will not have complete control over when your counseling function starts or stops, but you do have some control.

With regard to beginning a session, try to establish a certain atmosphere that indicates your desire to take the PWA (or whomever) seriously. For instance, you might want to ensure privacy and request that no interruptions be allowed for a certain length of time: family, visiting friends, or phone calls. Or you may want simply to adopt a special attitude by pulling up a particular chair and facing the PWA as if to say, "I'm here to help and I'm serious."

Ending a session is probably more important for the peer counselor, for s/he will not be likely to have an alarm clock that rings when the fifty-minute session is over. However, the counselor will want to codify the alternatives and wrap it up in order that the PWA not ramble on and on about his/her woes. Setting a personal time limit and sticking with it is not a bad idea. It gives you a frame in which to work to see some alternatives toward a resolution; it keeps you on track. Also, after several sessions, the PWA will recognize that when you counsel, you mean business. Summarizing is a good skill to use to curtail a session: "Okay, as I understand it, you have decided to talk to your doctor, first, about your inability to sleep; and if he has no suggestions, you have decided to forget it and not worry about it, right?" And, after you get confirmation, change the subject, remove your "business" attitude, and open the doors.

Sometimes ending a session can be difficult, especially when no clear-cut alternatives or resolutions have been reached. And yet, when you feel that the discussions have become mired, you will need to take action yourself. This may be uncomfortable to both you and the PWA, and this is when you will need to be tough, changing from the role of counselor to the role of friend: "John, neither of us has been able to see a way clear to keep you from being evicted tomorrow. I don't know what we are going to do. But I want you to know, for what it's worth, that I'm in there fighting with you because I love you. Somehow we'll make it."

▪ CONCLUSION ▪

The role of peer counselor is critical to the well-being of the PWA or PWARC. You play a special part in this tragedy, a part that is not particularly easy but that can be extremely fulfilling. Most of what you do is based upon common sense, empathy, and intuition. The one thing of which to remain constantly aware is the fact that only the person you are counseling can make the decisions that affect his/her life. Your job—and only when asked!—is to listen and reflect, define and clarify. To do more that this is to parent rather than counsel . . . and that is a completely different role.

▪ BIBLIOGRAPHY ▪

Borck, Leslie, and Fawcett, Stephen. *Learning Counseling and Problem Solving Skills (Instructor's Manual)*. New York: Haworth Press, 1982.

Carkhuff, Robert R., and Anthony, William Alan. *Skills of Helping: An Introduction to Counseling Skills*. Amherst, MA: Human Resource Development, © 1979.

Eagan, Gerard. *The Skilled Helper: Model Skills and Methods for Effective Helping* (2nd ed.). Monterey, CA: Brooks/Cole, © 1982.

Loughary, John William, and Ripley, Theresa M. *Helping Others Help Themselves*. New York: McGraw Hill, © 1979.

8

· STORIES FROM · THE FRONT: NUMBER 2 BILLY BURTON

BILLY BURTON

Billy Burton is originally from St. Croix in the U.S. Virgin Islands. He moved to Texas several years ago, where he became a decorative painter specializing in faux-marble finishes for furniture and other accent pieces. After his diagnosis, Billy became active in PWA activities nationwide, sitting as cochair and then as a board member of the National Association of People with AIDS and currently as a board member of the Lesbian and Gay Health Foundation. Prior to moving back to Dallas, Billy worked as the residence manager of the McAdory House, a temporary residence for displaced PWAs, in Houston.

I had asked Billy Burton, the PWA who was assigned to me in the Oak Lawn Counseling Center's Buddy Project, to write this chapter to explain how he worked with a buddy—a stranger in his life—and what he would tell other volunteers who are working with an AIDS patient they didn't know. What I expected was a list of dos and don'ts; what I received was a taped letter that says both more and less than I expected. Rather than

making suggestions of how the PWA and volunteer might work together,
Billy describes how the two of us worked together. Instead of editing this,
I have decided to leave it in its original form. The purpose is not to laud
my efforts but, rather, to show how important the volunteer can be,
certainly more important than he or she may ever realize.

—Ted Eidson

Dear Ted:

You asked me to talk about me, talk about my fears and apprehensions, how I opened my life to strangers (buddies, counselors, and others) and what I expected of them, how I dealt with my friends and family . . . it's difficult. Where do I begin?

Looking back over my notes, I see that I had a lot of fears in 1982 when I first got ill. First were the normal fears of someone recently diagnosed. Actually, I didn't even know what the diagnosis was at first. They were saying ARC and then, on the other hand, they were saying possibly AIDS. They knew so little. And I didn't know if I had any time to live.

I spent days at the hospital having tests run, and then going back the next day to find out that, "Yeah, there's something wrong here: You don't respond to your skin tests; your T-cell ratio is really low and the ratio is reversed. . . ." Each day was a new result from new tests but no real answers. The anxiety that one feels is just unbelievable. Often, I would go back to the doctor just to ask for something to calm me down, not from the disease itself, but from the doctor himself! There was nothing I could do but wait for answers and they didn't always come.

I got worse and I began to lose all the important things in my life: my job, my insurance, my friends, family, lover. Somehow I managed not to panic: My doctor went into panic long before I did, I think. All I know is that he looked at my back, saw what he thought were Kaposi's sarcoma lesions, stepped back, gasped, and said, "Are you insured? I want you to go to the hospital right away!" Of course, I was terrified.

When I was eventually diagnosed with ARC, I came home

and tried to call three close friends, all of whom lived in different cities. They were friends with whom the relationship held even if we were three thousand miles apart or hadn't seen each other in years. I called and found out that each had died or been diagnosed himself. It was terrifying.

I know that I was a real wreck. It was especially difficult dealing with Mom. When I asked her for assistance, her response was that she couldn't help any, that I had put myself in this situation and that I had got what I deserved for hanging around "dirty" people, and that those "dirty" people could just take care of me.

Then, Jonathan, my lover, walked out. Friends and pals just stopped being around, vanished. I had lost so much. And then, I started to push aside a lot of my friends, not because I couldn't cope with the situation but because I was beginning to realize that there were people I didn't need in my life any longer. I didn't want party friends; I didn't want to party and drink. I already knew that I had a sour liver, chronic hepatitis, and that I couldn't drink.

I was taking the opportunity to look at what I really wanted out of life, what expectations I had of myself. I found all of these negatives in my life and saw I needed more positives. The party friends no longer played a role in my life as I wanted it to be; and there were other people I was finding who I wanted in my life, who were supportive, who could reaffirm the positives I was trying to stay in tune with. But when you spend twenty-five years dealing with negatives all the time, you don't become a positive person overnight. I put a lot of work into it. And I knew that I couldn't do it alone.

I began by going to the PWA group sessions at the Counseling Center led by Vicki Morris. The first time was frightening, but as soon as I was there, I knew it was right. I needed good counseling and someone who would help me through these times. Group made a world of difference. Then, Vicki introduced me to imagery and visualization, Louise Hay's tapes. This was a new door opening for me; it helped a lot. It let me realize that I didn't have to be so bad after all.

I had heard some of the guys in group talking about having buddies and how beneficial it was for them; but they were worse off than I was. I had a lot of fear about meeting a buddy, or even asking for a buddy: It was very difficult for me. Opening up to a stranger has always been easy for me: I love to gab. But, opening *that* part of my life is pretty tough.

What I expected from a buddy was not very much, really. I just felt I needed someone to talk to at times. There were times I was lonely and there were times I needed to discuss my mom and family and so on. That's where you came in to help.

When I finally decided to ask for a buddy, I felt a great sense of relief: There was going to be someone coming by who would help and support me in some fashion. When you first called me . . . you were so positive. It was like, "Grab a pair of shorts; we'll just talk, get a bite, and go for a swim." Our phone conversation was so brief, but I was really excited knowing that we were going to your house for dinner. Just the fact of knowing that I was going to dinner with someone was such a delight!

I still didn't expect much, but at least I was going to meet someone who knew something about what I was going through, someone who wasn't a professional or another PWA. You were someone who had already made the decision that he wanted to be a friend to someone with AIDS, with someone who was going to be dealing with all of these fears and apprehensions.

When you arrived and I opened the door, you complimented me on the way I looked: It was overwhelming to me. I was looking in the mirror daily and seeing someone who had lost so much weight and had gone through so much muscular atrophy, wasn't built like he used to be, had bags under his eyes, and looked depressed. I could not conceive of anyone wanting to compliment this person. For months I had asked myself, "Geez, who in the world could possibly want me?" and "Is there hope?"

You and Vicki helped me in those early days to work through a lot rather quickly. I knew I had a lot of work to do, and I was aware that I could not do it alone. You showed me how destructive anger could be to me physically. You were constantly letting me know how good I looked: I needed to know I was not looking angry, depressed, stressful, to know that what I was doing was working. It was easier to look at myself in the mirror in the morning and see that I was looking better. I would take that attitude out and people would react to it: They began complimenting me again. So much of that was mental attitude! The fears would float away one by one; and as they floated away, a positive would come in to take their place.

There was a bond that we seemed to make: It was almost as if I had known you before. We could sit down and talk about things in common like the Islands, St. Thomas and St. Croix. I felt such incredible comfort. The simple fact that you would sit and cry with me when I cried and hurt with me when I hurt. It made it so much easier to get past those first stages and go on from there.

Do you recall the night we went to have Mexican food and came back to the house and put our feet in the pool so the mosquitoes wouldn't chew them up? We started talking about my mom and family and I just broke into tears. It was the first time, I think, that I really cried with you. I had recently lost both my dad and my sister: They had both died. Then Mom dropped me. You shared how you had had problems with your mother and how you dealt with them, relating them to mine with Mom; and you said to give her time, that she will come around. And if she doesn't, you said, write her off! You showed me that there might be a time right now when I just don't need her in my life and not to let her get to me when she comes at me with negatives, negatives, and more negatives. "Just love her," you said, "but remember that you are the most important person in your life." The more it is said, the more it sinks in.

That was an incredible step forward for me. I've come to realize that Mom is feeling very hurt by this disease. She's embarrassed and she is having to deal with a lot of her own fears about losing her son. She doesn't understand what's going on, and I don't have any real clear answers to give her. She doesn't have any idea what this is all about. All she knows is that this is a disease that kills people within six months to two years: That's where she's coming from.

As time goes on, she's coming around in her own way. She is still dealing with her fears and losses, and I still have to be understanding. I have to realize that when I asked her for help to pay my medical bills and she sent the silver flatware so I could set a nice table, that she was coming around in her own manner.

And, now she calls me to find out how I'm doing. A lot of times she still gets angry with me; but the more I "love her up," the closer the relationship becomes. I don't feed the anger and negativity with any of that any longer: I feed it with positives. Who can argue with love? Love heals. It's really important to me that she and I work through this and come to express our love to one another.

Crying that night made it so much easier to get past some of the old stuff and go on from there to focus on the immediate concerns: my health. I wanted to receive the best medical attention, naturally; but I felt that I was getting the runaround. My doctor would not call Houston to register me for the experimental programs for which I was qualified: He kept forgetting. You helped me work through the fears I had to deal with then by suggesting that I see another doctor, get a second opinion, maybe see someone who would be a little more along the holistic line.

By this time, I had a pretty good understanding that you were going to be as supportive as I required. You're a giver, but I don't think of you as a rescuer. At least you certainly punched me in the face a few times psychologically . . . and continue to do so! I appreciate that because I know that you care enough about me to do that. When I would get down and blue and start griping and complaining about my doctor, or about going to the clinic all of the time, or about having all the tests without getting any answers, you would shake me up and say, "Damnit, start doing some reading or go to another doctor!" You opened my eyes that I *could* go on with life. Sure, I was going to have to wait for a lot of answers, but that was no reason to loll around saying, "Woe is me." You got me to go out to the First International Lesbian and Gay Health Conference and AIDS Forum in Los Angeles. That opened my eyes to what I really wanted to do all along: to get back into working with people again, to use my psychology training. AIDS was something that was touching not only my life but the lives of many of my friends. We were all having to deal with death and dying, so many of us.

And then you got me to go to The Experience Weekend. That was an incredible step forward for me, going through that and seeing how many people had held on to so many horrifying experiences all their lives. I had never realized how good I had it! I had been living with this little, tiny thing, this "dis-ease" called AIDS for only a few months and already I was holding on to it, letting it run my life. The Weekend gave me the tools to change that.

Actually, I know now, having read my file, that the disease had been there for quite some time, that I had been diagnosed with full-blown AIDS in 1982! But they didn't tell me. It scares me sometimes that maybe no one knew then what was going on. Or was I denying the truth: I didn't want to know? Maybe it was both. Has not knowing played any role in my longevity? In any case, I have to look at whatever happened in the past as a real positive. To learn now that I have had full-blown AIDS for the last six years is pretty interesting. It starts up the old fears of someone recently diagnosed. Are things going to be worse than before? What does this mean? But it has also shown me a lot of things, like the fact that there really is a reason that I am here.

Thinking back, I remember that I had some apprehensions about meeting Gene, as our relationship developed. It seems we spent almost every evening together for several months! I kept thinking, Gosh, this guy's lover: What's he thinking? Was I interfering in your life? I wanted our relationship to develop into a relationship between Gene and me, as well. You mentioned talking with Gene about me and you said he might have some apprehensions about meeting me and dealing with some of his own fears. This was one of my biggest fears at the time: Was I going to screw up your life? Or, was I going to meet someone that I had so much in common with, that was so understanding, and that I could spend time with only to find that his significant other didn't want me around, or didn't like me, or was uncomfortable with me? Would I dare really open up and then lose you?

Would it come down to his meaning more to you than I? Those were real basic fears.

Our relationship has gone beyond those fears from early on so that you and Gene are virtual family to me now, the family support that I don't have from my real family. That may still come around in a while; but it's there for me now in the two of you. Even though we're so far apart now, I know you two are always there and willing to talk, happy to talk. You still support me in so much.

It's still pretty tough at times dealing with the death and dying: I think that is going to be an ongoing problem. I still have to deal with Warren's death—it still hurts a great deal—with John's death and with Howie's. There are all these people I would never have expected this to happen to. I find myself worrying sometimes about you and Gene. What would I do if this happened to one of you two? How would I react? How supportive could I be? You know I would always be there.

Dealing with my friends dying is the tough part. It hurts a lot, still. When I went to the Buddy Bereavement group with you, all of a sudden I realized how much grief I had been holding on to, and how much damage this swallowed grief could cause in terms of personal growth as well as physical health. We all have to deal with it, I know. It's part of life, regardless of AIDS.

And then I think about the loss of some of my friends and consider how long I have lived. I see people get diagnosed and die within two weeks! Sometimes I think it hurts more now than it ever did. Again I wonder why have I lived so long? Why are they going so fast? I don't know that I will ever come to a really clear answer to that. The only thing I have to go on is that there is obviously a reason somewhere. So I'm going to live my life to the fullest and be as positive as I can. And I can share those positives with others through the National Association for People with AIDS and the local coalitions around the country—Dallas and Houston. I can tap into others who have lived with the disease for a long time, and be able to help people who are newly diagnosed. We can be a positive example to show that we can live through this, that we can beat this. We have it within ourselves to work with our doctors, our friends, a metaphysician, acupuncturist, nutritionist, whatever it takes, to overcome this disease.

Working with AIDS makes me feel good because it allows me to touch someone else's life and see them go from near death to getting up out of bed, showing up at a meeting, and getting excited about having something to do. And they get excited about seeing people as sick as they were, or worse, who have bounced back, put their weight back on, and become healthy. They get excited about life and going on with their lives. They get excited about getting new jobs, going into social work, working in a service field, and so on. When we start the positives, we just get to watch them heal in larger and larger circles. This is what it is all about: This is what my life is about now.

What more can I say?

9

▪TOUGH LOVE▪

DAVID H. STOUT, A.C.S.W., C.S.W.-A.C.P

David H. Stout, A.C.S.W., C.S.W.-A.C.P., graduated with his Masters in Social Work from the University of Kansas. After four years of psychiatric unit work for hospitals in California and Illinois, he became Director of Social Work for the Texoma Medical Center in Denison, Texas. David became Director of Clinical Services for the Oak Lawn Counseling Center in Dallas in January 1987.

Tough love. The two words sound like a contradiction in terms, don't they? We are so used to thinking of love in romantic terms, more like a dreamy, marshmallowy kind of stuff. *Tough* love??? What's that?!

Consider the following true story of a little boy and see whether you can begin to see what tough love is all about. There was a ten-year-old boy living in a home for retarded and handicapped kids. Now, this little boy, Jimmy, was *both* retarded and handicapped: He was deaf and had leg deformities that prevented him from walking without his heavy, cumbersome, polio-type leg braces. However, in spite of his handicaps, he was attractive and had a very engaging personality. The staff in the home adored him.

Just a couple of blocks from the home was a fast-food hamburger joint where the staff liked to take the kids occasionally. Because it was so close to home, everyone walked. In this way, the frequent excessive energy of the kids got burned off just a bit.

When little Jimmy moved into the home, though, this put a damper on the hamburger outings. Jimmy walked much more slowly than the others; and when the group slowed down to Jimmy's speed, the other kids became fidgety and restless. "Going out" now exacerbated the very problem that it was to alleviate.

During one of these exasperating excursions, one staff member, in a moment of frustration, bent down, scooped up Jimmy, and began to carry him. This was much more efficient for the group's progress; and because this was a new game for Jimmy, he delighted in it. Both his cuteness and infectious laughter made the experience actually pleasurable for the staff member, as well. In the days to come, other staff members copied the solution and they, too, were delighted. Everyone was happy: staff, residents, and most of all, little Jimmy. Everyone felt good. Everyone got nice cozy strokes from everyone else. Sounds nice and neat, doesn't it?

In a staff meeting several weeks later, however, this solution was discussed. Someone pointed out that in just five or six years lil' Jimmy would be a teenager, well over six feet tall and weighing about 170 pounds. No one on staff would be able to carry him then. And what's more, he was missing out on invaluable exercise by being denied walking on the outings. His condition could conceivably deteriorate. The staff recognized that their solution, even though it felt good to them and to everyone else, was not the ideal one. They recognized that making Jimmy walk was in his own best interests.

Remember, though, that Jimmy was both retarded and deaf. Because of these combined problems, he had never learned to communicate. There was no way to tell him about the change about to be made, much less the reason for it. From his perspective, the change, when it did come, was sudden and without warning. There appeared to be no reason for it. His infectious smile and engaging personality no longer worked. No one would carry him. He had to walk with those damn heavy braces. It was as if he was being punished and he didn't know why. He cried. He bawled. He threw fits. Nothing made any difference. The staff would not carry him. They felt badly, too. A few tears flowed from their eyes, as well. No one was happy. It was a tough situation. The staff was learning about tough love. And little Jimmy didn't understand any of it.

What we can see by this example is that there is both a "soft" love and a "tough" love. The point needs to be emphasized here that neither is good nor bad, superior nor inferior, best nor worst, right nor wrong. Both have their places and both are, at times, inappropriate. The point is that *sometimes* tough love is required.

Now, just what does all of this have to do with Persons with AIDS (PWAs)? This manual is being prepared to help you folks out there in the trenches who are having to care for PWAs. That's tough. You're in a tough situation. Sometimes you'll need to be guided by tough love. This section is written to help you understand just what tough love is all about.

In order to understand tough love, though, we need to have a better understanding of how our minds work in the first place, how they work in most of us under normal conditions; and when we better understand that, then we can go on to understand how they work under adverse conditions.

You see, the mind is much like the body, a complex mixture of things that have different functions. The heart is shaped differently from the arms and performs different functions. Similarly, the mind has its functions—there are the feelings, the emotions, such as anger and happiness; then there is the thinking computer, which just deals with facts like how old you are and what $2 + 2$ are; and finally there is the conscience, which judges, nags, or nurtures us.

The story about little Jimmy gave us examples of all three of these at work. The feeling emotions were the first to respond to solving the problem. Kids were getting antsy, staff was frustrated, and Jimmy was tired. The solution was an emotional one: The staff scooped up Jimmy and carried him, to his delight. His change in emotion was contagious and the staff member began to have fun. The other kids relaxed and had fun, also.

The staff meeting a few weeks later, however, displayed the joint exercise of both judgmental conscience and thinking computer. The fact-finding computer did calculations about the future and recognized that the solution would not work for long. The conscience recognized that the solution would be detrimental to Jimmy. With these new data, the computer made a new decision and overrode the initial decision that had been made by only the feeling emotions.

These three different parts of our minds can be conceptualized as three different balloons or gas bags connected by a pipe (Diagram 1). Just like our lungs or our hearts, sometimes they are pumped up and sometimes they are deflated. In the story of little Jimmy, for example, the initial decision was based on everyone's feelings. The emotions part of our model was pumped up (as shown in Diagram 2). The later, revised decision was the result of the two other parts getting pumped up (Diagram 3).

One of the reasons that the initial decision about little Jimmy

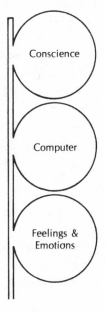

Diagram 1

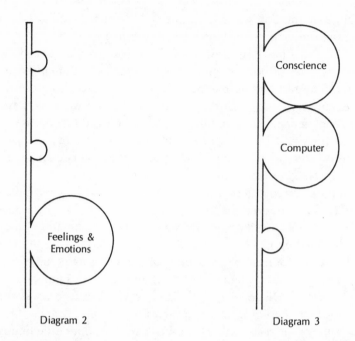

Diagram 2   Diagram 3

was emotionally based was because emotions are contagious. We
have all seen this. If someone is bubbly, it's not long before we
are all bubbly ourselves. Similarly, if someone is angry, everyone
else is soon aggravated. The tense emotional atmosphere in
which the staff person found himself with little Jimmy was contagious. The staff person became infected with the tension and
reacted emotionally to alleviate it. He fought fire with fire. As a
short-term solution, the choice was *very* effective. The problem
that emerged was the result of trying to use an effective short-
term solution to solve a long-term problem. In order to solve the
problem from a long-term perspective, an approach other than a
solely emotional one had to be utilized.

The PWAs you are working with are going to be full of
emotions—anger, depression, elation, fear, and God only knows
what else they might be able to dream up to feel! You will be
susceptible to these contagious emotions. You will undoubtedly
be infected by them and feel much like the PWA does. You will
react emotionally.

Not to worry, though. As we saw in the case of little Jimmy, *you*—unlike the PWA—can pull back and regroup. *You* can have a staff meeting of your own, even if it is just you having a talk with yourself! *You* can pull back from the disease—unlike the PWA—and find refuge in yourself or in others. You can redecide any decisions you make. You can use your computer and conscience to help guide you.

But, let's get back to the PWA for a moment. How come *s/he* can't? How come s/he gets off the hook?

To answer these questions, let's go back to our model. The model is one for healthy people. Just as our lungs ebb and flow, rise and fall with each breath, so it is with these three structures in our minds. However, we all have heard of people having collapsed lungs. When a lung collapses, this is not normal. The lung is in a pathological state. So it is with the PWAs and the pathological state they are in, both physiologically and emotionally. One or two of their "mental balloons" may (and probably will) collapse. The most frequent collapse will look like Diagram 2—that is, the PWA will seem very emotional.

But other variations are also possible. Some PWAs will collapse their emotions and pump up their computers. Such a reaction will be experienced by you as if you were dealing with a computer completely devoid of emotions. This is called an "intellectual defensive system."

The point here is simply that the PWA for whom you are caring is in an abnormal state of health, both physiologically and psychologically. You are not in an abnormal state yourself, although you may *feel* the contagion and *feel* physiologically and psychologically drained.

In order to maintain your balance, you will need to pull back and exercise all your resources. You will need to use your conscience, your computer, and your feelings. Although this sounds easy and simplistic, it won't always be so. You won't always have enough information. For example, complete the following: $5 + ? + ? = 10$. Obviously, there is not just one answer. The missing numbers could be 4 and 1 or they could be 3 and 2. You don't have enough information for your computer to solve the problem. Likewise, with your PWA, you won't always have enough information. For example, s/he may have been very weak for the past few weeks and now feels strong enough, s/he says, to drive himself or herself to the doctor's office. You're not convinced. Is s/he strong enough or not? Your computer doesn't have enough information. You will have to rely on your other mental parts (conscience and emotions—or intuition) in order to make a decision. You may make a mistake. So what? As we saw with little Jimmy, you can always redecide.

So what is tough love? Tough love is your utilization of all your mental parts to decide the who, what, when, where, and why of what you are doing, regardless of how it feels. Your PWA may be *very, very* angry at you, very sarcastic and hurtful. If you were to rely solely on your feelings, you'd be hurt, angry, and you'd probably leave. But then, who would feed your PWA? Who would bathe him or her? Who would change the sheets? Your computer and conscience will have to work together to recognize what must be done and what should be done—even though none of it may feel good.

On the other hand, your PWA may play helpless, much as little Jimmy did. You may feel very good to be so helpful, and you may find yourself doing everything for him or her, even those things s/he can do perfectly well independently! But s/he is so grateful, so kind; and you feel so good doing what you are doing, even though s/he should probably be getting up to keep limber. Again your tough love is needed here: your ability to stand back and fully assess the entire situation with your whole brain—with your conscience and computer and not just your emotions.

What is tough love? Tough love is getting the PWA out of bed and making him or her walk because that is what your brains tell you is needed. Tough love is leaving your PWA to go out for a movie and dinner, even though s/he wants you to stay, because that is what your brains tell you that *you* need. It's using *all* of you to guide yourself in tough situations and not relying on only a part of yourself, whether it feels good or not. That's a tough thing to do, because none of us wants to go against what we like to do or would prefer to do. You've got a tough job ahead of you. Using tough love will help you get through it.

▪ ACKNOWLEDGMENT ▪

The author wishes to thank and acknowledge Arlene N. Hess, another contributor to this book, for her inspiration and unwitting contribution to this chapter. In 1986, Ms. Hess presented the "tough love" portion of the Buddy Training. This presentation was videotaped and is now part of the Oak Lawn Counseling Center's video library.

10

· DEALING WITH · STRESS AND BURNOUT

E. TYRONNE HOWZE, M.A.

E. Tyronne Howze, M.A., received his under-graduate degree from Southern Illinois University, Edwardsville, and his Masters in Counseling from Conservative Baptist Theological Seminary in Denver. As one of the foremost AIDS counselors at the Oak Lawn Counseling Center, Ty was involved with almost every aspect of AIDS-related counseling, from soft aerobics for PWAs and PWARCs to training sessions for volunteers. Presently Ty works for the Shanti Project in San Francisco as an HIV counselor.

People get involved as primary caregivers for Persons with AIDS for many reasons. Some people do it out of a sense of civic duty. Some do it due to their love for humanity and a genuine desire to help. Others do it because they are family and feel a sense of love or obligation or guilt. And still others do it because they have a need in their own life that gets met by this kind of caring. Whatever the reason, it is of primary importance that you be aware of *your* reason for being where you are, for caring for a PWA. The more honest you can be about what is going on with you, the more you will find that you are able to benefit the person in your care.

What does self-honesty have to do with stress and burnout? Everything. Self-honesty is based upon self-knowledge and self-responsibility: knowing what is happening to you and taking responsible action in accordance with that knowledge. Being honest with yourself is the first and most important step in stress reduction. So, this chapter is about you!

Stress has to do with any change within a system that is induced by external force, or the emotional tensions and psychological demands that result from these changes. Simply stated, almost any change causes stress. The danger in stress arises when it is not bled off but is allowed to build up: More time is spent in coping than in living and accomplishing, which allows even more stress to build.

Burnout is the result of excessive stress. Literally the word means to be worn out by excessive or improper use or to be exhausted. Something (or someone) that is burned out is of little use to anyone. And yet this condition occurs frequently with the significant care providers for PWAs and PWARCs.

Before we go too far, let us look at a real situation and how stress and burnout affected the ability to give adequate care.

Ron had been diagnosed with AIDS for several months. He had not told his parents because he did not want them to worry. But his condition weakened so much that he was unable to keep his job and his apartment. As he could not find any other resources, he felt forced to turn to his parents.

His parents willingly took Ron in to live with them. But this meant that they had to deal with learning about his diagnosis at the same time they were required to reorganize their daily routine for Ron: The stress hit doubly hard.

When Ron first went home, everything seemed like a crisis.

If he sneezed, his mother would want to wash everything. In fear of contagion, they bought paper plates, cups, and so on for everyone to use. It finally got to the point where they got rid of the animals (birds, cats, dogs, etc.) not only because they might be a health risk for Ron, but also because his parents were afraid that neither of them would have the time to care for the animals and Ron, too.

Both parents started to avoid their neighbors and friends: They became tired of telling people, "Ron has cancer." In the process of isolating themselves, they isolated Ron, as well. They didn't want Ron's friends to visit because they thought the neighbors might learn that their son was gay.

Because his father had medical problems due to his excessive weight, Ron's mother took on the majority of Ron's care. Her stress mounted and began to become obvious. She was afraid to go grocery shopping during the day for fear that Ron might need her. She became unable to sleep, afraid that she wouldn't hear him in the night if he should call. When she slept at all, it was briefly and across the foot of her son's bed.

Things became progressively worse; and in the final weeks of Ron's life, the family, in exhaustion and burnout, turned to volunteers for help. His mother had become unable to maintain the pace of doing everything herself without adequate food or rest. His father's health had begun to deteriorate too, during this period as a result of the stress the entire family was undergoing.

Ironically, the volunteers met problems from the outset: Ron's mother had become so protective that she was unable to let go. She tried to direct everyone and would not allow anything to be said around Ron that might upset him. These volunteers were, however, able to give Ron the care he needed until he died.

Ron's parents are still recovering, not so much from Ron's death as from the devastation of their own lives. Because they had isolated themselves during Ron's illness, they have had to rebuild their social contacts and have not had friends to help them through their period of grief. Because they had given up their animals, they did not have even them for comfort. And the real tragedy is that a great portion of the stress might have been relieved if the family had recognized and taken responsibility for their *own* needs and sought help sooner.

This illustrates how important it is for you, as a caregiver, to be aware of the enormous amounts of stress you may be undergoing. It can render you completely unable to care effectively for your loved one without your realizing it. If you expect to continue being an effective caregiver, you will need to become attuned to what is going on within your own body and your immediate environment. If you are not attuned to yourself, how can you expect to be attuned to the changes going on within another? Self-honesty.

The areas to be on the lookout for within yourself that portend stress are:

> changes in blood pressure
> stomach pains
> anxiety attacks
> *depression*
> irritability
> poor relations with others
> increased drinking
> overeating
> retreat to sleep
> incessant watching of television
> obsessive reading

There are a number of other signs, but these should set the stage for you. The primary thing is to be aware of the *changes* in your daily emotional life patterns, such as those listed previously, which are signals that something is going on within you.

Of the preceding list, depression is often the most difficult to recognize within oneself. Stress and depression are not the same thing, but sometimes they may look the same. More often, though, stress is a precursor to depression. So let us define depression. You are feeling *depression:*

If you *feel* sad, irritable, despondent, discouraged, low, moody, numb, or fearful
if your *behavior* is withdrawn, shows a loss of interest in the usual things, has become procrastinating, or is incessantly weepy
if your *thoughts* are critical, negative, hopeless, and helpless.

More specifically, if you are experiencing five out of the following eight symptoms, you are definitely depressed.

weight or appetite loss
sleep disturbance (too much or too little)
fatigue or restlessness
loss of interest in routine or sexual matters
difficulty concentrating
feelings of guilt
thoughts of suicide or wishing one was dead
somatic (bodily) agitation

The reason that depression is so important is that it is often the precursor to burnout. Look over the signs of depression again; notice how each sign, if allowed to grow, could stop any and all activity. If you are the primary caregiver and your activity with your PWA slows to the point of stopping, if you *burn out,* your PWA is in jeopardy. It is that simple. Your objective as a caregiver is to help your PWA improve the quality of his or her life whether s/he lives six months or sixty more years. To do that requires you to become continually aware yourself: self-awareness.

It was agreed previously that anyone who takes on the role of caregiver will experience a major amount of change in his or her life and therefore some increased stress. The purpose of this chapter is not only to point out the signs but to give you the tools to bleed off stress before it becomes burnout. Only you can bleed off your stress: No one else is able to. It requires that you take responsibility for your life and daily habits: self-responsibility. The following list patterned from the *Wellness Workbook* give the steps to begin *today.*

As you read through the list, check off in the first column those that are presently under control, presently part of your daily habit. Then, begin working on integrating the unchecked areas into your life, checking them off when you feel comfortable with them. Use the second column several months from now or sometime in the future when you notice things getting really hectic or out of control. Again, check off first those habits you still maintain and begin reestablishing the others in your life as you are able.

SELF-RESPONSIBILITY

_____ _____ Get adequate sleep each night.

_____ _____ Eat a balanced nutritional diet.

_____ _____ Take moderate physical exercise at least three times per week.

_____ _____ Restructure lifestyle so that stress of daily routine is reduced or minimized. If boredom is a source of stress, engage in a more active lifestyle.

_____ _____ Know and accept your own limitations.

_____ _____ Know and accept the limitations of those around you.

_____ _____ Set both short- and long-term goals for yourself. Accomplishing short-term goals brings immediate satisfaction.

_____ _____ Engage in noncompetitive activities. Competitive activities increase tension. (Recognize that some tension is normal.)

_____ _____ Be aware of highly stressful situations. Do whatever possible to alter situations with potential for tension.

_____ _____ Remain calm.

_____ _____ Develop your own pace for living; avoid tasks that increase tension.

_____ _____ Plan and anticipate future pleasurable activities.

_____ _____ Take an occasional respite from responsibility as a temporary tension-reducing measure.

_____ _____ Use various methods of relaxation (e.g., visualization, meditation, biofeedback, etc.)

_____ _____ Be aware of your space at home. Make it enjoyable and pleasurable. Stark lighting and blaring radios and TVs increase tension.

_____ _____ Recognize when you are fatigued. It is a primary stress factor.

_____ _____ Channel emotional energy constructively. Release anger, disappointment, and anxiety by running, swimming, cleaning out your closet, taking aerobics, laughing, working in the yard, verbalizing, taking up a hobby, etc.

_____ _____ Avoid self-defeating thoughts.

_____ _____ Practice a habitual positive mental attitude.

_____ _____ Do not blame others or situations for the stress you feel.

_____ _____ Take responsibility for meeting your own needs.

Obviously this is an ongoing proposition and no one can be expected to accomplish all of the objectives on the list all of the time. So, the first thing recommended, especially for relatives of PWAs and PWARCs, particularly for parents, is to find a support system. It may come in many forms: from other family members to outside friends and/or neighbors, from groups of others working with PWAs and PWARCs to professional counseling or psychotherapy.

Often families caring for a loved one may find themselves isolated. Sometimes this isolation comes from fear: fear of rejection, ridicule, persecution, or any number of reasons. At other times it may be caused by the family's sense of obligation to the PWA or even guilt about the PWA. And if the PWA's condition is likely to result in death, the isolation could drag on for a year or more, becoming irreversible as friends and neighbors forget about you. The stress in caring for a PWA is likely to take its toll on you enough without adding a burden of isolation.

In addition to finding a support group, it's going to be very important for you to think through, or maybe rethink, your beliefs about death and dying (which are explored elsewhere in this book), as well as your beliefs about love. All of the buddies who have worked with PWAs and PWARCs, parents as well as non-related volunteers, have this introspection in common. Those who are still buddies have worked through it, examined their beliefs, learned to bend in the wind; the others who refused to examine and become reacquainted with themselves were those who burned out. When one chooses the path of a caregiver, one changes one's life. As one changes, one needs to be willing to reexamine the issues affecting one and reeducate oneself to the new life one is experiencing.

For example, when dealing as a primary caregiver, you may quickly come face-to-face with a person whose life patterns are totally different from yours. If you have not previously known that person, or not known him or her well, you will have to form some bonds of love in order to work together effectively in trust and respect. If you have known and loved the person previously, the love will have to be expanded to redefine new levels of trust and respect. What this means is that it will be very important for you to suspend any judgments you may have about the morality of the PWA in your care. Beyond what the lifestyle may have been (drug user, prostitute, homosexual, etc.), the PWA's morality will extend into every facet of his or her own daily life. The caregiver who stands in judgment of the PWA's attitudes and moralities, even lovingly, will lose the PWA's trust and respect. The caregiver who, on the other hand, allows himself or herself to be taken advantage of or to be run over will also lose the PWA. This is all part of the reeducation process.

Most caregivers who work on these aspects of self-knowledge reach a new definition of love called "unconditional love." This is a loving attitude that creates space for both the PWA and the caregiver, allowing each the space for growth and healing, while allowing that each might be growing and healing along different paths. Unconditional love is reassuring your PWA that you support him or her, while at the same time *setting limits on what you will and will not do.* Unconditional love is being there when you want to be there, and not being there when you don't want to. Unconditional love is finding a support system that will help you accomplish some of these things and taking the time to use it. Taking care of yourself is an act of unconditional love, both for you and for your PWA!

The objective for any caregiver is to help the PWA improve the quality of his or her life no matter how long or short it may prove to be. This is your objective, and it is one that will cause a number of changes in your life—that's obvious to anyone reading this book! It is the changes, however, that cause stress in life, and stress that is allowed to grow unchecked can lead to depression and eventually to burnout.

But stress is not difficult to bleed off *if* one is willing to maintain the self-responsibility required to recognize the signs of stress within oneself, and to further one's self-knowledge by learning and growing from the changes that AIDS brings.

▪ BIBLIOGRAPHY ▪

Benson. *The Relaxation Response.*
Kravette. *Complete Relaxation.*
Kübler-Ross. *Death: The Final Stage of Growth.*
————. *On Death and Dying.*
Ryan. *Wellness Workbook.*
Schaefer. *Stress, Distress and Growth.*
Selye. *Stress Without Distress.*
Shaffer. *Life After Stress.*

(Full bibliographical information may be found in Appendix F.)

11

· STORIES FROM · THE FRONT: NUMBER 3 PETER

RODNEY HOLCOMB

Rodney Holcomb continued with the Buddy Project after Peter's death, as chairman of the Education Committee that is responsible for all of the buddy training and ongoing buddy education sessions. In 1987, Rodney resigned from the Buddy Project in order to go to work for the newly formed AIDS/ARMS Network, a nonprofit organization funded in part by a grant from the Robert Woods Johnson Foundation. As a Care Coordinator, he is responsible for locating and coordinating services and resources throughout the county for Persons with AIDS or ARC.

You know, it's funny writing about Peter almost a year after his death. At one time, all you had to do was mention his name and volunteers immediately knew who you were talking about. The Buddy Project has grown and other Peters have come and gone, but this Peter will always hold a special place in my heart. What's funny now is realizing that at one time I would never have even thought that!

My involvement with the Buddy Project began in November, 1985, the last training session in which the Center's founder, Howie Daire, participated. At the end of that day, a special request was made for volunteers to work immediately with a man named Peter living in the Oak Cliff section of Dallas. I volunteered and waited for a call that never came. At the time, it really bothered me that no one had called; but soon after, I began feeling that being a buddy might be more than I had bargained for, anyway. So, I simply waited to see what would happen.

Shortly after Christmas, I received a call asking me to attend an organizational meeting the next Sunday. At this meeting, I was told, "You're going to be a cell leader: How does that sound?" For the next twelve months, I managed a group of eight to twelve volunteers who worked with PWAs, as I was soon to do.

As a cell leader, I was brought up-to-date on Peter from one of the volunteers who was paying for his apartment. Peter had been found bedridden in an apartment in Denton, Texas. He was unable to prepare meals or provide for any of his daily living needs; in fact, he was found lying in his own urine and feces, unable to get to the bathroom. Some concerned individual called the Oak Lawn Counseling Center, and Peter was moved into an apartment in Oak Cliff. A second indigent PWA, John, was chosen to move in with Peter to help him with his meals and needs and to watch over him. It was moving to know that people cared enough to assist someone to this extent.

Within a couple of weeks, I was a member of a five-man buddy team that worked with Peter through the progression of his disease. (There were another thirty buddies who volunteered to work with Peter, but he ran them off!) I vividly remember driving to Peter's the first time on a cold January day. It was my first case and I was nervous. Time dragged and everything seemed to work against me. When I arrived, I couldn't get the fence gate open. When I finally did, a dog came charging at me from behind the house, causing me to freeze in my place, which in turn allowed Rusty to jump on me and cover me in mud! When I finally made it to Peter's door and opened it, I was hit with this incredible heat and the odor of an old, unaired, gas-heated dwelling. Indeed, things were not as I had imagined they would be.

There is nothing, I suppose, that can really prepare one for this first meeting. But as a volunteer, one knows that one is there to provide comfort and assistance and to help lend as much dignity as is possible with this disease. One realizes that it is a meeting of two distinct, unique individuals and that each situation should be met without expectations. I reminded myself of this as I entered Peter's room.

When I first saw him, he was still bedridden and probably weighed about 115 pounds. I walked in and sat on the end of the bad, grinned, and said, "Hi, my name is Rodney; I'm with the Buddy Project and I'm going to be one of your new buddies." Peter looked at me, looked the other way, and focused on me again. Silence. Finally, he said, "I guess you think it's real nice to come down here from fashionable North Dallas and help the 'Poor AIDS Patient' down in Oak Cliff." Then he threw the bedsheet to one side, exposing his thin nude body, saying, "This is what you got!"

I thought to myself, This is not starting out like I wanted.

Not knowing what else to do, I smiled and told Peter, "You're going to catch cold if you don't cover up; and besides, you don't have anything that interests me, anyway!" Then I got up, surveyed the apartment, and cleaned the kitchen sink. When dealing with Peter got too heavy, the buddies headed for the kitchen: Some cursed; others smoked; I cleaned the sink. And he did have the cleanest sink in South Dallas!

Peter was an angry individual. He was angry at the world, angry at having AIDS, angry that his brother would outlive him, angry at his mother for disowning him six years previously when he told her he was gay, and angry at God. In 1980, Peter had met a man and taken him to his apartment. During the middle of the night, the man bludgeoned Peter with a claw hammer and stole his pride and joy: his oversized, Texas Cadillac. For three days, Peter's friends telephoned, but there was no answer. They went by and knocked, but there was still no answer and no car. Worried, someone finally broke in and found Peter in a pool of dried blood. It was apparent from the stains that Peter had tried to get to the phone before collapsing. He was taken to the hospital. The verdict was that he would not live, or if he did, only as a vegetable. Peter surprised them all (as he did us, on numerous occasions) by making a complete recovery, though the right side of his head would always have a caved-in area.

This story helps one to understand his intense desire to live, as well as his anger toward his family who deserted him when he needed them so desperately. Additionally, Peter had bargained with God when he was in the hospital—if God allowed him to live, he would stop smoking, drinking, and having sex, and become a good Christian. God did; but within a few years, Peter had developed AIDS. The promises he had made and kept religiously were torturous for him, but only once did his resolve fail, and he took a sexual partner for a night. So, Peter was angry at God for what he saw as God's retribution, and angry at himself and guilty for what he saw as his broken vow to God.

Maybe it was Peter's anger that gave him the strength to live. Or possibly it was his fear of dying and meeting a vengeful God. He became a member of both Metropolitan Community Church (a Methodist offshoot) and Church of Christ. Or it may simply have been that Peter lived to drive his huge black Cadillac, which was located and returned to him, the only thing remaining from his previous life. Whatever the reason, it took five of us to minister to his needs. Two Steves, Bob, Greg, and I provided care in the evenings in addition to grocery shopping, laundry service, and transportation to and from doctors' appointments. As Peter was afraid of being alone, the five of us depended on each other heavily for support, especially toward the later stages of his illness.

For a while, Peter took an upswing and became surprisingly stronger, able to walk a bit and to go to church. During these times, he could be fun and charming. But as winter moved into spring, he began to deteriorate, and again we bore the brunt of his anger. I remember one night fixing him a can of vegetarian vegetable soup (the only one he would eat, though he wasn't a vegetarian) according to the directions, using one can of water. I sliced an apple and put it on a plate with the soup and crackers. Like many AIDS patients, Peter's appetite was nil due to the medications and the normal loss of taste the disease can cause. I had hoped that he would eat a bit more than just the soup that night.

When I took him his tray, Peter just played with his soup, not eating anything. Suddenly he looked up and said, "You can't make soup right, can you?"

"Excuse me?"

"You put a whole can of water in it," he accused. "I'm not eating this!"

So, I told him I would fix another can, went to the kitchen, drained the water, rattled the pan, reheated the soup, and took it back in. Peter managed to eat five or six spoonfuls and a couple of apple slices, evidently pleased with the "new" soup.

I started working with Peter in January and worked with him until he died in the first week of May. The last five weeks were extremely difficult on all of us. Unlike a lot of the buddies, we had not had problems dealing with family members, as they simply didn't come around. At times, we wished they would, because we could have used their support, lots of it.

As Peter declined, spring was in full bloom and the abundance of life was evident everywhere. In Peter's room, there was a growing smell of sickness, stale air, and sweat: death. Like many AIDS patients, Peter would get chilled to the bone, and have the gas heater turned up full blast as he shivered under a pile of blankets. The room stayed at 88 degrees, making the smells oppressive. As his body began decaying, the odors became more cloying.

Leaving Peter's room and walking outdoors was always a shock. It was such an obvious juxtaposition of death on one side of the door and life on the other. I saw life and death as two separate entities with no common bonds. At the time Peter was dying, my sister-in-law was expecting her first child: I was to be an uncle. And once again, I was struck with life on the one hand

and death on the other! Why this was so startling and confusing to me, I couldn't understand until months later: I was grieving for Peter. I had grown to love this dying, angry man!

Peter continued to decline in health even after there was no health left to decline from. Toward the end of April, Greg took Peter to the VA Hospital, where they spent the entire day, as was common, waiting for doctors and test results. A doctor finally pulled Greg aside and said, "I want to know what you guys are doing. Peter should have died two weeks ago. None of his major organs are functioning at anything near acceptable levels and his blood is toxic!"

Peter was eavesdropping on the entire conversation and heard the doctor tell Greg that he wanted Peter to stay there at the hospital. When Peter heard this, he lost all motor control and slid out of the wheelchair onto the floor, such was his fear of dying in the hospital, alone. It took some doing, but Greg managed to get Peter back into the wheelchair and to act strong enough for the doctor to allow him to return home.

Peter lived almost five weeks after that, a testament to his willpower. The last two weeks, he was comatose, but he never closed his eyes. It was as if Peter was afraid that if he closed his eyes to sleep, he would never awaken. So the five of us kept his eyes moist with eyedrops and waited for the end. We were exhausted, mentally, emotionally, and physically.

And then one Saturday morning, after I had left Peter's when Todd, the home companion, arrived, I headed for the Counseling Center. There was a buddy support meeting that morning that I needed to go to. I was just about ready to toss in the towel and tell everyone that I couldn't take it anymore, when I received a message to call Todd. I left the meeting and called quickly, expecting the news that Peter had slipped away. What I heard instead was a frustrated and angry Todd saying, "Peter is causing me a lot of problems. I've tried to change his catheter, but he won't let me; and he won't let me empty his urine bag!"

"What?" I asked. I seriously doubted what Todd was saying, for Peter had been comatose for over a week, not talking, not closing his eyes, not doing anything.

"Peter's raising hell about my changing the urine bag!" he yelled. And in the background, I heard Peter scream, "That's a damn lie!" Peter was alive again. I was in shock. I talked to Todd and calmed him down, and then to Peter and got him settled by telling him exactly what Todd was trying to do. After walking them both through the catheter and urine bag change, step by step, I went outside to sit in the sun, numb, completely burned-out. Another buddy came out to see how I was doing. I remember saying to him, "I was raised having the answers, but I don't have any more answers now." I was past the edge of what I could take.

That night I dreamt about Peter. In the dream, I was driving down Central Expressway and saw Peter stranded on the roadside by his big black Cadillac. He was waving for help, so I pulled over. He came up to my window and said, "My car has broken down; can you give me a lift?" I replied, "Sure," and we drove on down the highway. After a few miles, Peter said that he had to get off at the next exit. I replied that that was fine because I needed to go in the other direction.

That was how the dream ended; but when I awoke, it all made sense. As a volunteer, I was there to help someone who was unable to help himself. That was what I did when I stopped and picked up Peter in the dream. I helped him get to where he needed to go; and when we reached that spot, Peter let me know that he had to continue his own journey, in his own direction, different from mine. I wasn't there to save him, cure him, or make him better; I was there to make sure he was as comfortable as possible and could die with dignity.

I also learned that his death was his own experience and that he was in control of that situation. I had been afraid that his being in a coma, refusing to shut his eyes, was a sign of his struggling against death. In the dream, I allowed his death to be his own, knowing that he had reached his own level of acceptance. He reached this level by struggling with it for months. It was not what healthy people want to call it: "giving up." There's a big difference. Peter was still afraid of death, but he had accepted it of his own accord. He stayed in control of the situation. I realized that he was a brave man and I felt privileged to be working with him.

The five of us buddies all met different needs for Peter. Bereft of family, Peter directed a lot of his love toward Steve and was always expressing it to him. He would tell Steve often that he loved him and wanted Steve to come to work for him. Steve would jokingly ask, "Well, Peter, how much do you get in Social Security?" Peter would tell him, and Steve would say, "Well, I'm a lot more expensive than that!"

To some extent all the other buddies became Peter's overtly loved family. Peter would make a point of telling them how much he loved them. And Peter demanded love from all of us as his due. Sometimes, he would tell the buddies, "If you loved me, you would do this for me because I'm dying." To this extent he was like a child saying, "Mom, I need this new bike; it will make me feel better." But, like a child, Peter needed discipline and boundaries set for him. This became my role. Maybe I represented his father who had died so many years before and whom Peter had not been able to know as a grown man. Whatever the reason, Peter never would tell me that he loved me, as he would the others. After a while, I just tried to accept this as part of my role.

The night before Peter died, Bob, Steve, and I stayed with him. Peter had slipped back into his coma several days before, and we knew he would not live long. We stood huddled at the end of the bed looking at his frail seventy pounds. We would talk about Peter and begin to cry. As Peter wanted never to be alone, we stayed. Even though he did not respond, we constantly let him know we were there. We told him that we loved him, that he was protected, and that it was safe to let go.

Bobby had been sitting on Peter's bed and after a while, I took his place. Perched on the restraining bar of the hospital bed, I cradled his head against my chest and washed his forehead with a cool damp cloth. I kept talking to him, reciting the Lord's Prayer, and telling him that it was all right to let go, that everything had been taken care of. I then told him, "Peter, I really do love you; do you know that?" He heard me, for he wrapped his little finger around mine and squeezed tightly. He held on to my finger in the same way for the next hour and a half until I started to get up. Then he held on even tighter. I asked, "Peter, are you trying to say something?" and I leaned down to hear him in case he could talk. He squeezed my finger one more time and whispered, "I love you."

When I went home that night, I felt closer to Peter than I ever had over those long months. I was totally aware of him. Even his death smell was on me still. I showered and fell into a sound sleep. I awoke at three-thirty that morning and stared at the clock for the next hour before going back to sleep. Later that morning, Steve called me at work to tell me Peter had died quietly sometime between three-thirty and four-thirty.

My nephew, James, was born hours after Peter died, and suddenly, deep inside, it made sense that death is as much a part of living as life. For me, death was no longer separate from life but part of a continuum. Peter had died on this physical plane while another life had come into being. It was part of spring.

12

· THE HEALING · PROCESS CALLED GRIEF

ARLENE N. HESS, M.ED., AAMFT, L.P.C., CADAC

Arlene Hess is a private psychotherapist in Dallas who specializes in substance-abuse problems and death and dying psychology. She has volunteered her services to the Buddy Program of the Oak Lawn Counseling Center's AIDS Projects, where she has trained prospective buddies in the issues relating to death and dying, and where she continues to facilitate bereavement groups for buddies who have lost their PWAs.

We have all been around another person who was grieving and we can remember how we reacted to their grief, what effect their grief had on us for better or for worse. Conversely, we have each grieved about something in our own lives, so we know the raw energy that grief unleashes. With AIDS, as with many terminal disease situations, the stage is set for concentrated grief. The AIDS patient grieves, his family and friends grieve, the caregivers grieve; but each person grieves at a different level. Everyone dealing with the patient will eventually have to deal with his own grief as well as with everyone else's. To further complicate matters, each person's grief process, being totally subjective, is almost always out of sync, off pitch, and on a different level from everyone else's. The potential in this kind of setting for faux pas, hurt feelings, and lost tempers is extremely high. How one person's grief is processed will have a direct effect on the health of everyone within that sphere of influence.

Ironically, the stage is set exactly opposite to how anyone would have it. Given our druthers, most of us would shelve our grief and that of others until after the crisis (if not shelve it forever). But that's not the way it works. So what we must do instead is to learn about what grief is, how it works, and what it seeks to do for us. We need to understand its process so that we may stop interrupting its course, both in ourselves and others. We need to come to recognize its signs so that we may understand where we and others are coming from. Most importantly, we must come to understand grief as a healing process to be supported rather than fought. We are in the midst of the AIDS crisis to lend our healing powers, our caring, however we may. Understanding the grief process correctly will provide us with information to release an abundant amount of energy for healing.

▪ DEFINING GRIEF ▪

Grief is an automatic, richly complicated, multifaceted human phenomenon. It is a process of movement, a process of moving through the pain of loss-trauma toward a new higher level of consciousness. It is a simultaneous process of healing and learning.

Traditionally, we have misunderstood and resisted grief by trying to ignore it. We saw only pain and the loss. We chose to cling to our love-objects as if they were guaranteed permanent, to swing forever in mid-air on a trapeze without a net to catch us when change occurs . . . and change will occur. Every relationship ends and we lose our love-object, be that a person, place, job, home, or be it an attachment to a particular rigid image: ourself or another as a youthful person, dancer, mother, and so on. Everything human changes; all are ephemeral; all human relationships end! Change is reality. It has been said that the suffering that comes from loss is due to the ropeburn of holding on to that which no longer is. Grief, then, is the process that allows us to let go as it heals the ropeburns. And it is something more.

To understand grief, we need to look at its counterpart: love. Loving is not an act of will, nor merely an emotional response. Though it contains both those elements, it is far more. To love another person, place, or thing involves a multilevel investment in the loved "other" with emotional, cognative, physical, and spiritual elements called "bonding." All love is bonding and vice versa.

Every love experience, every bonding experience, is subjective, individual, and unique. The love we experience for any two anythings is not the same: The bonds that tie us together happen at various levels and with varying intensities. When the love-object is lost to us, we experience the pains of the various bonds being severed. As the pain of loss is felt, we must allow and release this pain so that healing can be allowed to happen at the affected levels. Grief like love is multileveled and multifaceted.

WE CAN NOT CURE
             BUT
                   WE CAN HEAL.

It was stated earlier that love transcends the physical and emotional, and often has a spiritual dimension. When this love is lost, it is the spiritual level that does not cause pain: As the other levels of severed bonding heal through grief, the spiritual level remains intact, clear and beautiful. If we think of the spiritual level of love (regardless of what it is we love) as being something beyond our own humanness, something on a higher level, then it will be seen that when we allow it, the grief process brings us to that higher level. This is the reward of grief. To try to avoid and shelve grief not only mires us in the pain, it also delays us from reaching our deserved reward.

The grief/healing process is very personal and subjective. For example, the length of time and order of emotional stages differs from person to person, and within one person, from loss to loss. With regard to AIDS, the grief process can be expected to be especially complex, for all the persons involved will be experiencing the crisis from their own unique perspective, therefore focusing on their own specific loss. Persons with AIDS (PWAs) and Persons with AIDS-Related Complex (PWARCs) will frequently be experiencing their loss of health, jobs, home, friends, and independence. Additionally, they are having to face what Freud called "the big fear," loss of life. If the PWA's image of self is strongly tied to the physical (*I* am this body; *I* am this life!), the loss can be felt as total.

Family members may be grieving for the loss of their own expectations: The grandchildren that are not to be, the football trophy never won, the lost companionship. Medical personnel have the grief of not being able to cure, of "letting another person die." Much of this is anticipatory grief for what will not be in the future.

GRIEF IS NEITHER SIMPLE NOR OPTIONAL.

Anticipatory grief makes the final grief less intense and helps toward a more rapid healing. It's healthy and should not be met with condemnation ("Stop crying: He's not dead yet!") but with encouragement and understanding ("Would it help you to talk about it?" "What you are feeling is natural; I understand.").

Possibly the most important aspect of anticipatory grief is

that it opens the doors to closure. By giving us the chance to project into the future and see the loss before the fact, we are granted time to be *real* with the dying person, to say the things we always meant to, and, perhaps, to share on a deeper level than previously. Regardless of our beliefs in a hereafter, there is a need within humans to reach a conclusion with what they begin: And this lifetime is ending! Closure is goodbye to what is now to be ending. It allows the grief/healing process to work more smoothly without becoming snarled in "unfinished business," all the "if onlys" that continue to haunt us.

More often than not, people enter the grief process carrying old, unresolved griefs and guilts. When we enter the AIDS arena and the grief process begins, we might see in ourselves and others (including the PWA or PWARC) areas of intensity that do not seem relevant to the situation. Normally, what we are seeing is "unfinished business" from the past that is shirttailing on this new grief issue. Knowing this might be enough to help sort out the old stuff from the current experience and relieve some of the current anxiety. Also, it underscores how important it is to our future emotional health to bring an emotional closure to our current experience of loss so that it doesn't pop up again in the future.

▪ PROCESSING FEAR ▪

Ideally, the completed healing process of grief would have let go of whatever fear is created in the void of the loss. For both the PWA and the PWARC, the fear most basic and easily identified is death. The PWA or PWARC faces his or her personal, immediate death; and s/he may seek to overcome that fear by reaching an understanding of what life and death are in the cosmic view of things. More than the PWA, the PWARC also faces the fears associated with *not* dying, of living a half-life, energetically crippled by constant ailments and diseases and prone to contracting a terminal disorder at any time. The PWA may tend to ask questions such as, "What is death about?" "What was my life about?" "How can I still come to know my God?" The PWARC may view death as being farther away and may ask questions such as, "What is or should my life be about?" "What changes can I make in my life now?" "How can I make this life worthwhile for me, humankind, and my God?" Personal health is generally not the immediate concern of the family and loved ones, but their fears are just as real. Being caused by the death of another, their fear tends more toward questions such as, "How can I live without this person I love?" "Will the pain ever stop?" "Why were they taken from me?" "What is the point of life without them?" "If there is a God, why does He take the good people?"

> **HEALING IS LETTING GO OF FEAR.**
> **HEALTH IS INNER PEACE.**

This facet of the healing process may push a person to ask spiritual questions and look at personal religious beliefs. The resolution of the process may be metaphysical. If the healing process is completed, if the fear is released, then an acceptance of the inevitable—almost a surrendering—will frequently be experienced, and usually a sense of deep peace.

Also, many of us expect that time in and of itself will heal the wounds of loss. We add to our own pain when we fall into this trap. It is for this reason that it is so important to understand the grief/healing process. Knowing where the PWA or PWARC is, and realizing where we are with our grief in relation to theirs, we are able to offer our caregiving abilities on a wholly different level. Knowing where family and loved ones are emotionally will allow us not only to assist them but also to be a buffer between them and the PWA, between their levels of anticipatory grief and the PWA's current grief. Finally, this knowledge allows us to protect ourselves from the emotional fireworks that are by-products of grief/healing, even when the fireworks are our own!

• VISUALIZING THE •
PROCESS

A simplified model of the grief/healing process looks like the diagram below.

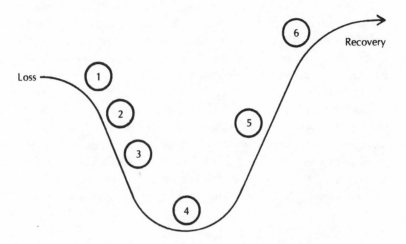

1. Denial: "This isn't happening to me. The doctor has mixed up my blood test with someone else's."
2. Anger: "What did I do to deserve this?" "Get away from me: You can't help me!" "I know now: There is no God!"
3. Bargaining: "I was wrong in my life: Let me live, God, and I promise I'll . . . ." "If I eat everything on my plate, I'll gain weight and get my health back."
4. Depression: (crying, lethargy, insomnia, withdrawal form everyone and everything, a total giving-up) "Why mess with anything; I'm going to die anyway. It's hopeless."
5. Acceptance: new energy, interest in the *now,* concern about caregivers and family, appreciation for life and others.
6. Hope: extension into the future, commitment to something beyond self.

Though the examples of each stage are presented from the PWA's viewpoint, the stages themselves are universal in their description of grief, regardless of who is experiencing it or why. By reading back through the list and substituting examples more akin to a person's own situation, one will see more clearly how the model runs.

Once the "dip" has been worked through—the feelings and issues faced, expressed, and dealt with—then the thrust to recovery takes place. We know we have successfully completed our work when we can recall the loss of the love-object without having an accompanying emotional reaction. In other words, we can remember that Jim died last year, but we don't feel a tremor, headache, nausea, fear. We just have a mental recall. It has been put in our memory system, but our emotional reactions have dissipated. The person who successfully completes his or her grief work emerges stronger for the experiences and able to live on a richer, deeper level of life than ever before.

Knowing the model allows us to monitor another person's

The way is *not* clearly marked!

grief or our own. But it does not allow us to make any of it happen faster: "No thanks, I'll skip the depression part; I had some of that just recently." The problems with models, regardless of how complete, is that they are deficient. Just like road signs, they don't tell you everything that will happen on the trip, and they do not prevent one from having to go back and forth over the same road more than once.

Unlike the nice models, the stages do not flow in neat, orderly progression. They are confused, frequently happening several at a time, repeated, and hopefully digested. Often in working with a PWA, we feel that he has finally reached an acceptance of his death, that things are getting better. And then, just when we are ready to relax, the PWA will drop a bomb such as, "You know, I really don't think I do have AIDS," and suddenly we're back at the beginning of the curve. But then everything works and *movement* towards a resolution, healing, and inner peace is continued.

• COMPLICATED • GRIEF

What is dangerous is when the process becomes mired. This is "complicated grief." It is similar to a wound that closes without its having healed: It becomes infected, more painful, and potentially poisons the whole human system. With the PWA, the process often stymies in the denial stage. The PWA may deny that he has the disease at all, thereby potentially infecting his or her sexual partners or creating and giving birth to an infected child. Or the PWA may deny that he has lost his health and run himself into the ground trying to do what he used to be able to do, tiring himself out and opening himself to a plethora of opportunistic diseases. A PWARC may have a tendency to become enmeshed in the depression stage, unable to move in any direction, pulling himself into a downward spiral mentally, which has been linked to lymphocyte suppression, which can allow the occurrence of more opportunistic diseases. And we have all witnessed the pitiable person who never recovered from a loved one's death: their lives are spent aimlessly, living ghosts who weep and walk the floors late at night.

Regardless of the stage at which the process is interrupted, complicated grief is dangerous. If the process is not allowed to go on its normal course, it will go underground, so to speak, and fester, causing a variety of psychosomatic illnesses and more misery than the original loss did. As caregivers, we need to be on the lookout for such complications. Though we are not able to speed up the process, just allowing that it's okay to feel and express all of these feelings may be enough to keep the process moving along.

While we are in the midst of the AIDS arena, it is almost impossible to know when someone's grief process has become mired. There are no time parameters for any of the stages and no guarantees that a particular stage will follow another. Though there are no clear-cut signs, there may be some hints. A person may deny a stage completely or jump through it too quickly: "I'm not an angry person, this doesn't apply to me." The hint may be just the opposite, that one or more stages themselves seem to become severely exaggerated. Or a person may change his social behavior, becoming completely introverted or completely extroverted. The most telltale sign, however, can be more easily seen in people other than the PWA, manifested in headaches, unexplained gastrointestinal problems, and other physical symptoms.

As caregivers, we are working toward healing, achieving an inner peace with *all* persons involved. We help a person through complicated grief with the same tools we use in uncomplicated grief:

Being receptive: willingly entertaining new concepts
Maintaining physical presence: touching and hugging
Practicing permissive listening: allowing the time
    for them to talk through their stages, to voice
    fears, and so on

Giving what is needed along with what is wanted:
  tough love engenders strength
Keeping contact with the loving part of the world:
  providing a homing beacon to be seen by those
  at sea
Knowing our own theology (or atheism or
  agnosticism): owning up to it and sharing it
  peacefully

If it seems that the process has become mired, speaking honestly of that concern may be all that is needed to break the deadlock. Otherwise, the caregiver needs to seek professional help for the person in grief.

Ironically, it is the PWA whose grief process is working against the clock and whose disease symptoms hide the signs that hint of complicated grief. Because of this, and in order to have a touchstone for our own health, the caregivers are always strongly urged to seek out support groups for themselves. They need people who understand the problems and issues and who can act as sounding boards and sources of insight. It is not a good idea for a caregiver to assume that he is seeing a complicated situation clearly: He's probably not! At this point, what is needed is an objective, knowing *other.* Grief work is largely an individual experience that needs social facilitation, tender "others" who can provide a nurturing, safe atmosphere.

■ PERMISSION TO DIE ■

The model above and the grief process that is developed herein place the active portion of healing on the grieving person. The people near a person in grief play a passive role in the process: supportive, reflective, and so on. With a terminal patient, though, one active moment is often required of the rest of us at some existential point: giving that patient permission to die. Without that permission, it is extremely difficult for the PWA to make it to the stages of acceptance and hope. Without the permission, they will become completely mired at the bottom of the curve, or they will try to struggle upward carrying tons of guilt: "If I accept my death and stop fighting, I'll let my friends, family, and loved ones down!"

Western culture teaches us that death is an enemy to be avoided. Social Darwinism teaches us that the fit survive, which is to say that those who die are the unfit. Religion teaches us that suicide, passive or active, is a sin. And yet, if a PWA is expected to reach a resolution of the death and dying process, the "bad" has to be taken out of death.

Often the reality of death is reconciled by the PWA much more quickly than by family members or caregivers. The PWA has already had to rethink many of his or her cultural viewpoints. She or he may have realized, for instance, that the youth culture is not all it is cracked-up to be when s/he, the youth, is dying. He or she may have realized that sex and beauty are somewhat shallow as meanings of life. And s/he will have begun to realize that the *illness* s/he suffers so painfully, increasingly, and terminally is the real enemy. He or she will begin to see death as a friend, especially if s/he has processed the other grief issues. All that s/he will lack at this point in order to move through acceptance into hope is permission from the people s/he loves and respects. Too often, we, the loved ones and caregivers, are the block to progress; too often, we impose our limited thinking on the PWA's struggle for peace.

Giving permission to die is difficult for us. We, too, are bound by cultural values and by our personal religious beliefs. Furthermore, we as caregivers are acutely aware how the will to live affects a person's health: We will fight tooth and nail for a person to have a "positive attitude." With AIDS especially, positivism is the only medicine we have found to combat the various diseases effectively and unremittingly.

But as we watch a friend or loved one waste away, watch the pain become less bearable and more frequent, we wonder why. We watch them valiantly trying once more to muster the strength to fight off some bug that a healthy one-year-old would have no trouble conquering, and we weep! We say to ourselves, "Let him die, let him be released from his misery." But, on the surface, we

say to the PWA, "Don't stop fighting yet; don't give up now."
The PWA senses our confusion and this usually confuses him or
her. Certainly this is not healing.

There is that existential point at which we have to stop being
cheerleaders and humbly accept the reality that it is up to us to
assist in surrendering to death. But how? First, we must be attuned to understanding that the time has come. Then, we must
be able to step outside our own emotions so that our minds are
more clearly in the *now* with the PWA. Finally we have to be
willing to own up to our own feelings as genuinely as the PWA
has. The result is a dual affirmation: "I want you to live a long
life and I'm really going to miss you. I'm very angry about this!
But, also, I know that you are hurting so much. I don't want to
be selfish: I want to help you do what's right for you. What are
you feeling? What are you thinking? What can I do to help?
Where are you in this process?" If we can be this clear and open
about our own feelings, perhaps by example we will be able to
give PWAs the courage to tell us as much as possible how the
experience really is for them.

Somewhere along the line, the dying PWA may have
reached a new respect for death, a respect due an equal if not a
friend. When that happens, there will come a shift in attitude, a
level of acceptance not previously evident. And likely, there will
be hints that death is no longer frightening. It is not possible to
say *exactly* what it is that will alert the caregiver to the fact that
the PWA is seeking permission to die. But if we can quiet our
own conflicting ideas and provide a space of acceptance for the
PWA, usually s/he will share with us and we will know.

Two tools discussed earlier come into play heavily at this
juncture: receptivity and permissive listening ability. If the anten-
nae are up, you will hear the question; and if you have your own
life and death philosophies in place and maintain contact with the
loving part of the world, you will know what to say and how to
say it: It will be completely natural and healing. You will know
when the time of closure has come and you will join with death
in assisting your friend on the unending journey, whatever you
may consider that to be.

And yet sometimes, no matter how hard we have tried to hear, no matter how open we have been, the existential point either doesn't come or we weren't there when it did. Or maybe the PWA never reached that peaceful stage. Whatever the case, there can be a closure from our side, which is needed for our own healing process. Holding a hand or simply maintaining eye contact, you might think silently, I love you and I give you permission to be whatever is best for you.

> DR. PIETER V. ADMIRAAL, DUTCH ANES-
> THESIOLOGIST AND LEADING PRACTI-
> TIONER OF EUTHANASIA AS QUOTED IN
> *NEWSWEEK:* "I SAY TO MY PATIENT: 'I
> WISH YOU A VERY GOOD JOURNEY TO
> AN UNKNOWN YOU HAVE NEVER
> SEEN!' "

The involvement of a caregiver does not end with the PWA's death. Oftentimes, there has been a bonding with other caregivers and with the PWA's family and friends. There is the simple fact that at the PWA's death, the grief process continues for the survivors. Hopefully, the caregiver has experienced some anticipatory grief while working with the PWA, and has been able to work through a lot of the stages before death. Not only does this make the final goodbye easier to process, it also indicates that something big has taken place.

· THE JOURNEY ·

Caregivers—often complete strangers—who volunteer to work with the dying are often asked why they put themselves in such a position, how they can stand the pain and suffering. The answer is that there is something that happens between the dying person and the caregiver that cannot be put into words. It has to do with sharing the most intimate experience of a person's life: death. It has to do with unconditional love, the love that flows between the caregiver and PWA that makes no judgment calls. It has to do with the closure that takes place between a dying person and another. There is an incredible sharing that takes place when people die consciously (whether or not they have processed their grief), and you are there to share in the farewell into the new journey.

The caregiver has given time and love in ways that people see and respect, even if they do not fully understand. But the caregiver has received "gifts" from the dying person: trust and love of a kind rarely experienced, and the dying experience itself. It is all of this and something more that the caregiver receives.

In trying to explain what it was about, one volunteer whose PWA had died offered the following analogy that he referred to as "The Journey."*

Imagine helping a friend on a journey to a remote monastery perched on top of a mountain. As you begin your trip, the path is fairly clearly marked and the goal easily seen in the distance. But as you approach, the monastery is often obscured by the tops of trees in the forests through which you pass. And you say, "If only we could get out of this woods, we would be able to see the monastery again and see where we're going." And the woods thin and for a while the monastery is seen until it is again obscured by an outcropping of rock or possibly the clouds and mists that sometimes settle on the mountaintop. And as you continue the climb, the path fades and much is accomplished by guesswork. You call on your friend for

*The analogy, here entitled "The Journey," was originally given to me by a longtime supporter of the Oak Lawn Counseling Center, Joe Fleming, when trying to explain why he had agreed to become a buddy. Though it has been expanded upon for this writing, its sentiment is genuinely Joe's.

help: After all, this is his trip and he should know what he's doing. But he has become older and more decrepit and relies more on you moment by moment.

Things get worse. You lose the path, and you are tired and hungry. It's not fair! This isn't your journey: It's his! But, he can not proceed alone and you can't leave him to rot on the side of the mountain while you return to the warmth and safety of home. So, you find a new reserve of strength, enough for both of you, and you continue up the mountain, for now it is your journey, as well.

You look at yourself anew and find that you have grown older, become more mature like your friend, and you accept this as part of the mutual trip. And in accepting your role as guide, you find that you are guided, that your friend, whose legs have crumpled beneath him by now, offers you wellsprings of courage and hope. You drink deeply, for you realize that if either of you are to make it to the top, it will need both of you guiding and supporting the other in ways constantly changing and unimaginable.

One day when you least expect it, the heavy cedar gates of the monastery are suddenly dead ahead. The trip had become the whole purpose, it seemed, and the monastery forgotten. But there it stands: Your friend's objective has been reached. The door opens to admit your friend and, as if you had performed the ritual many times before, you hand your friend over the threshold. The door closes, and you stand there numb, alone, bewildered.

Out of habit, you continue walking. It doesn't seem to matter in what direction, for each of the possible paths lead back down from the mountain.

The trip down seems easier than the trip up was. The mountain holds few surprises, now, and there is ample time to sit and ponder before reaching the valley below. And somehow in reviewing the trip with your friend, its moments of desperation and fear are overshadowed by the times of giving and accepting, of sharing and journeying together. Memory of the monastery fades and in its place stand crystal images of points along the upward trek. There was the time when you picked him up and carried him across the rocks when his strength failed. And there was the time when you slipped and lost your grasp, but he held you up and supported you with the power of his mind. There was something special in those moments, something, which if you could string all of those images together in just the right order, that then, maybe then, you would understand.

As it is, you return to the valley a different person, quieter and stronger, knowing only that you have been a part of something . . . holy. This friend, this stranger, shared with you his most personal possession, his death. And though you can't quite comprehend its true value, you find yourself hoping that you will have the ability to fully experience and share your final journey with another wayfarer to whom you can pass on crystal images.

▪ CONCLUSION ▪

Deep gratitude and celebration are the order of the day for those of us who are called together to assist in this challenge of the AIDS crisis. For the PWAs, the families, lovers, and volunteers, the challenges are incredible. The suffering, remember, is found only in our refusal to let go, only when we refuse to go through the pain and move to the other side. We get through by going through. The rewards are wonderful: the joy and blessings that come from extending the self beyond its own comfort zone; the knowledge we gain of life and death; the love that is lost and found again on a higher plane; and the areas of awareness that are opened. Grief is a healing process to be welcomed and not feared, for when it is allowed to go its own course unobstructed, it will fill with wonder the void that the loss created.

The whole of life
Without any exception
May be an act of worship
If man chooses to make it so.
—John Woodruff

13

·PASTORAL·
CARE

REV. TED KARPF

Father Ted Karpf is an Episcopal priest and rector
of the Church of St. Thomas the Apostle in Dallas,
which is the site of Buddy Training and numerous
AIDS awareness training and caregiving sessions.
Father Karpf has worked with more than two hundred persons with AIDS and ARC and their families. He was a founder of the AIDS Inter-Faith
Network in Dallas, which now boasts ninety religious leaders who have agreed to be on call for
pastoral counseling for AIDS issues. Likewise, his
parish was the first in Dallas that welcomed and
ministered to Persons with AIDS and their families.

The crisis of AIDS has brought forth a desire by many to offer
some kind of care or support. Because of the nature of the disease, which usually ends in death, many assume that pastoral care
is needed. This may not be true for all people with AIDS or their
families. What do we mean by pastoral care? This is a vital question for us to consider. Then, we need to see how it may be
extended by *anyone* who is willing to be vulnerable and loving.

First, it is very important to consider what issues are present
and what struggles are inherent in the process of living with

AIDS. In facing AIDS (or any other terminal disease), one must finally come to terms with issues regarding the *value* as well as the meaning of life. Because there is a vast array of diseases that can inflict untold suffering on the person with AIDS and that make living itself a punishment, it is simply not enough to cling to life at all costs. In fact, with this disease, the prospect of clinging to life may be more oppressive than letting go.

However, when the conversation regards the comparative merits of death and life, a larger discussion of soul matters will invariably be present. Questions about God and life, sin and death, reward and redemption are very likely to be raised: "What is my meaning and purpose in the larger scheme of things?" "What is my ultimate destiny?" "How can a loving God do something like this to me?" and "Am I being punished for sexual or societal [e.g., drug usage] sins?" These are the questions we all raise at some time or another: They are questions that reflect our faith as well as the faith of those who suffer. In a word, they are universal questions not unique to AIDS, and must be seen in the context of living rather than of death. The difference between the well and the terminally ill is that of staking the totality of one's existence, one's faith, on the answers derived from experience to date. The well have next year's experience in which to test the tentative answers about meaning, which the terminally ill do not have.

The first step in caring for the souls of persons with AIDS is recognizing that disease and death do not create new issues about faith; rather there is an urgency to resolve old issues. Perhaps more significantly, there is a realistic need to get on with the issues of faith, life, and meaning in an way that makes sense and can be made harmonious within the life of one who is struggling with terminal illness. The question looks like this: "Am I living and facing my death in a way that is consistent with the faith that I hold?"

The danger for the caregiver is to rush in with an answer in order to allay the verbalized fears of the stricken person, or in order to allay one's own fears of the inadequacies of one's own answers! The bottom line is that we all have to find our own answers in this crisis, as we do in all of life's chances and changes. The answers can only be shared when we are asked to do so. Otherwise, we may be trying to fill the gaps of someone else's struggle and thereby depriving them of the integrity of their own convictions.

The next step is to recognize that we are all struggling for meaning and value. Few of us want to die, and all of us need to be loved. To care for souls, we must address these issues first in ourselves and then in those for whom we care, for in facing our own issues, we will be better equipped to accept the facts of that struggle in another. What makes this so doubly difficult is that persons who have an HIV-infection are ordinarily within the first thirty-five years of their lives, a time characterized by establishing outward or external career, vocational, and life goals and dreams. In the natural stages of human development, there has been little time to deal with the internal or soul issues of spirituality, faith, identity, and wholeness.

Indeed, all of these are being addressed, albeit incompletely, in the mere act of living; but by and large, the first half of a person's life is spent in establishing the external order so that s/he may have the material on which to reflect in the second half of life. For someong living with AIDS, all of this is going on at once against the unknown time line of a ticking clock. Hence, the very fact of AIDS and the mere existence of the normal human struggle for wholeness create an extraordinarily high level of intensity.

A mitigating factor against finding a fulfilling resolution of these conflicts of living and dying is the disintegration of one's social, domestic, and economic identities. The person with AIDS is losing all of the visible signs of living successfully, the symbols of integration and fulfillment. Added to this are the radical physical and mental changes due to both the treatments and the diseases, as well as the routine life/death issues. The result is a highly stressed person among other highly stressed people under tension-inducing conditions. To provide soul support for a person with AIDS, it is imperative that we realize that we are living out a variety of struggles in the midst of great stress. The overpowering need of both the caregiver and the person with AIDS is for grace/acceptance. Both need to experience this grace/acceptance through experiencing grief over loss fully and well; through the release of all the "could haves" and "should haves" and "only ifs"; through the release of identification of self from achievements, behaviors, successes, and objects; through experiencing trusting and loving relationships; and finally, through the discovery of hope.

Hope may be seen in a variety of ways by a variety of people. Writing in the *Texas Hospital Quarterly,* Dr. Oliver VannOrsdall, AIDS Chaplain at Parkland Memorial Hospital, describes hope's many aspects. Hope, he writes, may appear as an attention to finding a cure or to beating the odds, as staying focused on life and denying the reality of death. Hope may turn also toward a desire for a quick and painless death, minimum suffering and maximum alertness, personal control over the long haul, or a limitation of the burdens on loved ones and family. In the last stages of life, obvious hope appears in looking for an afterlife: be it life eternal or reincarnation. Hope is also expressed in funeral and estate planning, even in the disposition of one's earthly remains. The need to hope is universal. The reality is that we usually do not know how the questions of hope will be answered: They are, after all, matters of faith.

To the one who would be caregiver and soul-friend, these questions must be answered within. Hope is how we choose to cope with life and death. Making decisions is the way given to us to express our fundamental beliefs about living and dying. The way we express care for the person with AIDS is to encourage, support, and even challenge the individual to make as many of the decisions as possible throughout the process. Again, the only real answers are the ones each of us find in our own way.

However, the way one accepts life and one's answers to life is to achieve some level of personal acceptance, acceptance of self as well as acceptance of another's answers! Indeed, the issue of acceptance is paramount. In Christian terms, we call this, grace. Grace is not only the choices we make but also the freedom to choose, or even not to choose. If we truly value life, then we will value the choices and nonchoices that another makes. Affirmation and acceptance can best be experienced in our surrender of our needs to those of another. Our message to the person with AIDS is that this person is loved and accepted. Depending on our own faith, tradition, and experience, we may well perceive this as God working through us in the life of the one who is afflicted. More poignant, we may also come to find the one who is afflicted has become a vehicle of grace in our lives, as well.

Finally, with regard to seeking professional assistance or ordained soul care for the person with AIDS, it must be a matter of choice for the person with the disease. Seeking care and counsel for yourself as a potential caregiver or soul-friend is a matter of choice, as well. It is important to examine your feelings, prejudices, biases, thoughts, attitudes, and behaviors regarding sexuality, drugs, disease, death, life, and faith. No one comes to these issues willingly but, rather, with a certain sense of struggle. Change is inevitable with or without AIDS. Facing life and death, hope and acceptance are part of life's agenda in any circumstance. AIDS simply has become a means of getting focus more immediately. Soul care will go on with or without the church or organized religion. The person who cares for another with this disease simply need recognize that while the moment and situation are unique, the issues, struggles, and needs are not.

Some clergy, ordained or lay, may or may not be sources of comfort and support. Let your instincts guide you. Test out your hunches. Have no fear in testing those who would care or provide a service: They are trained to expect it. And if they are intimidated by your questions, then you are probably well advised to look for help elsewhere. Likewise, do not assume just because your particular tradition or faith-expression has historically been judgmental with regard to life and death questions, sin, drugs and sexual issues, disease, and guilt distinctions that there is no one who will listen and provide support or comfort. Time after time, the universality of this most human struggle— to find hope, acceptance, and peace—brings out the best in people. That, too, is a gift of grace and a sign of God's presence.

▪ SECTION III ▪

PRACTICAL MATTERS

14

• HOME CARE OF A PWA •

LIZABETH STEPHENS SHELBY, R.N. AND TARA ROWE, R.N.

Lizabeth Stephens Shelby, R.N., graduated from Pacific Lutheran University, Tacoma, Washington, with a B.A. in English. She later earned her Associate Degree in Nursing from the Maine Medical School of Nursing in Lewiston, Maine. She currently works as a nurse with the AIDS Prevention Project of the Dallas County Health Department.

Tara M. Rowe, R.N., received her B.S. in Nursing from East Tennessee State University. Having worked for several years in medical intensive care, she is presently employed as an R.N. supervisor-auditor.

Care of a terminally ill loved one at home can be a meaningful and rewarding experience; but anger, frustration, and stress also accompany this type of situation. And when that loved one has AIDS, there may be a fear of the illness itself. This section about the activities of daily living is to give you straight forward information that will help you approach home care in an informed, comfortable manner. Knowing how it should be done will also give you confidence to confront a hired aide if it appears their care is inadequate.

As the caregiver, it is important to pay attention to yourself and your feelings *first*. If you don't, you won't be able to take care of anyone else, especially someone who may be totally dependent. To do this, allow yourself to take a break; and if you need help, ask for it. There is nothing wrong with not being able to "do it all." Find out about home health aides, visiting nurses, or any services offered by private or state agencies. To care for *your* feelings, find a friend, relative, or therapist with whom you can discuss the difficulties of caring for someone at home.

It is very important to involve the PWA in his own care. Discuss needs with him or her, how s/he feels and what s/he feels like doing for himself or herself. When you are involved with physical, hands-on situations with your PWA, state what you intend to do, step by step. This not only avoids fear on his or her part, but allows the PWA to help you to the extent s/he is able. Confront your PWA when s/he is demanding too much, especially when s/he could be doing something independently. In fact, s/he should be encouraged to do as much self-care as possible. Many feelings—guilt, pity, and even a sense of martyrdom —often make us want to do everything when a family member or loved one is ill. It often gets to the point where it is the doing that becomes important rather than the person. Sharing feelings will make home care easier and will prevent the silent suffering that comes when the caregiver feels too much is expected, and the PWA feels merely like an object to be moved and manipulated.

Be honest. Be open. Ask for help. Outline your expectations of the PWA; allow him or her to express expectations of you. When the basic communication is open, it gives you both an opportunity to explore your relationship and share your love.

What follows is written in an easy-to-follow outline form. When the need arises, you will be able to flip to the section you need at that time and perform your duties confidently, one step at a time. Read through the sections now, and practice each until it makes sense to you and you feel comfortable. Learn what to do before it is required.

I. **General Assessment**

   A. Before starting any care, identify the PWA's needs, capabilities, and limitations for that day. A person's physical condition can change dramatically, becoming better or worse, from one day to another.

      1. Observe how the PWA is moving about in bed: easily, with difficulty, or in pain.
      2. Talk to the PWA about how he feels.
      3. Assess what the PWA may do for himself.
      4. Ask the PWA what he would *like* to do for himself.
      5. Involve the PWA in as much of his own care as possible.
      6. Be flexible: The situation may have to be reassessed during the day.

   B. Do not do for the PWA what he can do for himself.

      1. Encourage the PWA to do as much for himself as possible.
      2. When the PWA starts a task, watch him perform it.
      3. Offer help when he appears to be having difficulty reaching a certain area or is tiring.
      4. Don't set time limits: Be patient.
         a. It may take the PWA longer to complete a task than it would you. This is okay.
         b. Help the PWA to work to his maximum capabilities, but learn to identify when he truly is tired.

   C. Give the PWA support and feedback about how he is doing.

      1. Be honest and direct.
      2. His efforts should be recognized.
      3. Offer encouragement and praise.

Fear of contracting AIDS often makes people overreact when caring for a PWA. This is displayed by refusal to touch the PWA or by using elaborate protection with gown, mask, and gloves. To combat this fear, it is necessary to remember how the AIDS virus is transmitted: blood to blood; semen to blood; vaginal secretions to blood. It is not airborne, so a mask is not needed for self-protection. It is not transmitted by casual contact, so a gown and gloves are not always required. When you are doing hands-on care and are likely to contact a PWA's body fluids, such as urine, feces, open wounds, or any secretion that may be contaminated with blood, a gown and gloves are advisable. To enter a room, to talk, or even to feed a PWA, gown and gloves are not needed. When they are used, it is also important to explain to the PWA why they are being used, so the necessity of these precautions is clear to both parties. By understanding the infectious process and by not overreacting, both you and the PWA will be more comfortable.

Hugging and kissing are safe. Touching is safe. And both are therapeutic.

The real danger is to the AIDS patient and the germs *you* may take into the room with you. It is the patient's defenses that are depressed; *he's* the one that needs to be protected. Consequently it is important to remember to wash your hands frequently and before hands-on care. If you have a cold or a cough, wear a mask to protect the PWA and remember to explain why you are wearing protection.

The information that follows is possibly extracautious; but they are also the common-sense guidelines one follows with any ill person. The only additional precautionary steps here have to do with protecting yourself from the patient's blood, as there is the miniscule possibility of becoming infected through cuts or abrasions one gets on one's hands and arms. There has never been a documented transmission by this route to a home caregiver, but there is the possibility.

II. Infection Control

A. AIDS transmission: blood to blood, semen to blood, vaginal secretions to blood.

B. Protect yourself from a PWA's blood and other bodily secretions, especially those that may contain blood. These include urine, feces, vaginal fluids, and open wounds or sores.

C. Basic guidelines when providing hands-on care:

   1. Wear gloves when handling blood-soiled items, body fluids, excretions, secretions, or materials that may be contaminated with these fluids.

   2. Clean any surface that has become visibly contaminated with blood with a solution of 1 part bleach to 10 parts water.

   3. Wear a coverall gown or garment, long-sleeved, when clothing or skin is going to be exposed to a PWA's body fluids. There is no need to gown-up otherwise.

   4. Remove gown and gloves in the patient's room. Throw gloves away in plastic sack with other disposable items. Tie the sacks and put in the garbage. Wash coveralls in hot water and bleach.

   5. Wash hands in hot water before and after working with the patient. Use soap. This protects the PWA from the germs you carry into the room with you, as well as protecting you from the germs you may pick up from the PWA's fluids.

Appendix C has some further information and hints about protecting everyone from germs. You may want to read all three articles when you have the time.

One of the most common complaints that medical professionals hear is that of back trouble resulting from the improper use or overuse of back muscles. Perhaps the most basic, yet the most important subject to be covered in this chapter is the use of good body mechanics. Some of these activities will feel awkward at first because you may be used to doing them incorrectly; it is like learning a proper golf swing or a new dance step. As you read the hints that follow, practice each one; they will form habits that will keep you from tiring as rapidly as you might otherwise.

III. Body Mechanics

A. Keep your weight balanced directly above your feet. When your center of gravity is above the base of support, you can keep your balance and stability with much less effort.

B. Wear practical shoes and keep your feet apart. A sumo wrestler maintains better stability than a high-fashion model!

C. When necessary to increase your stability, such as when lifting a heavy box from the floor or helping a patient out of bed, keep your center of gravity low. Do this by bending at the knees and keeping your back straight, rather than by bending at the waist. Lifting is easier by bending the legs and using those muscles rather than the back muscles.

D. Place one foot in front of the other when pushing or pulling a heavy object, such as when moving a patient from the middle toward the side of the bed. This allows you to apply more force because you are using your leg muscles instead of just your back and arms.

E. Turn your whole body. Don't twist at the waist to pick up or move any object. This lessens the risk of back injury.

F. It is easier to move an object on a level surface than to move it against the force of gravity. For example, if the patient has a bed with a raisable foot or head, it will be easier to move him when the bed is level. Likewise, slide an object across a smooth surface rather than lifting it: Slide the patient rather than trying to lift him.

G. Hold close to your body anything or anyone that is to be moved, or stand close to whatever it is you are moving or transporting. You can't offer any real support if you are an arm's length away.

H. Use your own body weight to help in lifting or moving. For instance, when you help a patient stand, use the weight of your body to rock back, counterbalancing the patient's weight.

I. Move slowly and smoothly when handling a patient. This requires less energy, allows for better control, and keeps the patient feeling secure.

J. Remember that it is easier to pull a patient than to push him.

Now we are ready to begin the hands-on work. You may wish to mark this place in the book with a bookmark or paper clip so that you can find these sections easily in the future.

First, we will go through the steps for moving a patient, both to position him in bed and to assist him out of bed. It's easy and it doesn't require the caregiver to be either large or strong. Just follow the steps.

IV. Activities of Daily Living: Patient Transfers

   A. Assessment

      1. Evaluate the PWA's strength and movement capabilities.

      2. Set appropriate limits, but allow the PWA to do as much for himself as possible.

      3. Discuss how the transfer is to be made. If unfamiliar with the PWA's condition, ask how he is usually moved from one place to another and learn what areas of his body to be careful with.

B. Principles

1. The goal is to achieve a safe transfer without injury to the PWA or yourself.

2. Do not lift or pull using your arms and back muscles alone. Position your feet to use leg muscles and for balance.

3. Keep your center of gravity low. This is accomplished by keeping your feet apart and knees slightly bent: Be a sumo wrestler.

4. Use your own body weight to counterbalance the PWA's.

5. Pulling a person is easier than pushing him. Assisting a person who is under his own power is easier still.

6. Slow smooth movements require less energy, offer better control, are safer, and don't alarm the PWA.

Let's start the patient transfers with learning to roll the patient onto his or her side. You will need to know this later when you learn to make the bed with the patient in it. Then we will show you how to scoot the patient up (or down) in the bed.

C. Techniques for Raising up in Bed and Rolling onto Side

1. *Rolling onto side.* Place PWA's right arm across his chest to roll him onto his left side. (Reverse to roll onto right side.)

2. Stand on the side of the bed toward which PWA will turn. Reaching over the PWA, untuck the draw sheet (a flat sheet, folded in half, tucked in over the fitted sheet under the patient's hips) and pull it snugly against the PWA's back. Rolling up the excess of the sheet, grab this and use the sheet to roll the PWA toward you. When performing this maneuver, make certain your knees are bent,

rocking forward to grab the pull sheet and rocking back, pulling the sheet up taut and toward you to roll the patient.

3. Steady the patient on his side by placing a pillow behind his shoulders and upper back. Pull the lower shoulder out a bit so that all of his weight is not on this bony area.

4. If needed, place another pillow between the knees and reposition sheepskin (often used under feet or hips to avoid chafing).

5. *Raising up in bed.* Have the PWA lie flat on his back. Lower the bed (if a hospital bed) so that the surface is flat.

6. Position the soles of the patient's feet firmly on the surface of the bed. If the patient is able, have him grasp the headboard or side rails to help himself up.

7. Keep your feet at a wide stance, lean close to the PWA and cradle his shoulders and head in one arm. (Or you may wish instead to slide both hands and arms under the patient's hips, bending at the hips and knees.)

8. On the count of three, the PWA pushes with his feet toward the head of the bed while you assist in sliding either his head and shoulders or his hips.

9. If the PWA is unable to assist at all, two people are needed to move him up or down the bed. *Do not attempt to do this alone.*

10. Both people roll the draw sheet up until their hands are near the patient.

11. With feet apart, knees bent, elbows bent, count three and rock from the back foot to the front foot, shifting the weight toward the head of the bed and sliding the PWA upward at the same time.

Knowing how to move the patient around on the bed will make your tasks easier and help keep the patient comfortable when s/he is too weak to help her/himself. When the patient is stronger, it assists in getting them out of the bed.

D. Technique: Moving PWA to the Edge of the Bed and Helping Him Sit

1. Supporting his neck and shoulders with one arm, pull the PWA's head and shoulders toward you to the edge of the mattress.

2. Make certain that all tubing is out of the way.

3. Next, move PWA's legs to the same side of the bed. (His hips are still in the center of the bed, so PWA is now in a curved position.)

4. Slide both arms under the patient's hips until your hands cup the PWA's hips on the other side.

5. Bend your knees and tighten your abdominal and back muscles.

6. Pull the PWA's hips toward you until they are at the edge of the bed.

7. Stand beside the bed facing the headboard with one foot in front of the other. Place one arm under the PWA's shoulders and the other around him. Have the patient place his arm nearest you around your shoulders and to use his other elbow to press into the bed.

8. While you straighten your knees, rock back, pull the PWA up and toward you. The PWA should help by pushing himself up with his free arm and lowering his legs over the side of the bed.

9. Steady the PWA in this position for a few moments in case he becomes lightheaded or dizzy.

If the patient is strong enough, getting out of bed can be a welcome addition to the daily routine. It will make the patient

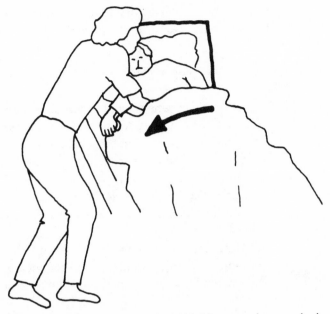

Place arms under patient's hips. Pull PWA's hips toward you and edge of bed.

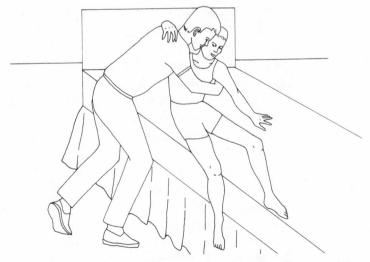

Pull PWA up and toward you. Gravity pulls legs downward, which raise trunk to sitting position.

feel less like an invalid, while allowing you the freedom to change the sheets or whatever with complete freedom.

E. Technique: Helping the PWA Stand and Move to a Chair.

1. Place the chair, wheelchair, or portable toilet one or two feet from the side and head of the bed at a 45-degree angle to the bed. Lock the wheelchair or wedge a standard chair so that it will not move as weight is leaned against it.

2. Have the PWA place his feet firmly on the floor, well under him and slightly apart, as he sits on the side of the bed.

3. Standing close to the bed in front of the PWA, bend your knees, feet apart, and put your foot nearest the chair behind you and turned out slightly to steady you.

4. Face the PWA, placing your hands firmly around his rib cage. (Or put your arms around his waist or under his arms, clasping your hands in back, whichever is the most comfortable for him and the sturdiest position for you.)

5. Press your knee against his knees or your foot against one of his feet to brace and balance him as he begins to stand and to keep him from sliding.

6. If desired, have him place his hands on your shoulders for his sense of balance, and rock him forward to a standing position.

7. Pause a moment to make certain that the PWA's legs are "locked," supporting him.

8. Holding the PWA in the same grasp, pivot him to the chair by the side of the bed and lower him into it, bending at your knees rather than your back, and sliding the PWA down your body. The PWA should grab the arms of the chair first in order to help position and lower himself.

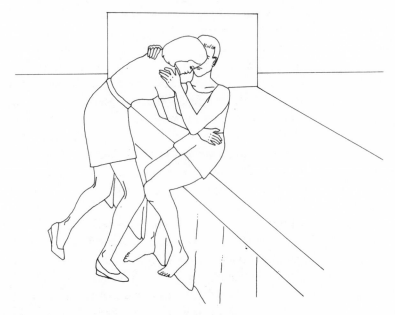

Push knee against knee of patient and rock to a standing position.

Sometimes a patient feels strong enough to move, but the body may not be totally cooperative. A bed-bound person is likely to have weak legs that can give out completely and unexpectedly. Knowing how to control this situation can save both of you bruises (or worse). Practicing it with someone can keep it from being traumatic for anyone should it ever actually happen. Slips and falls should not be something extra to worry about; rather they should be something for which one has been prepared.

F. Technique: Helping to Walk; the Controlled Fall
   1. Following the preceding steps, help the PWA to a standing position and stabilize him there.
   2. Keeping his arms on your shoulders, and putting your arm around his waist (or grabbing hold of his belt), pivot toward him so that the two of you are

facing the same direction and he is at your side supported by you.

3. After he has become steadied and you feel comfortable with your balance, move forward. The PWA should be moving under his own strength and you should only be offering balance. Stand close to him, but do not carry his weight.

4. If the patient begins to fall, you should assist his fall by lowering him to the bed, chair, or floor. Use your body as a slide if possible, pulling the PWA toward you and lowering both of you to a stable position.

5. If the patient begins to fall while walking across the floor, pull the patient against your chest with both hands, allowing the PWA to be supported by you. If you are unable to steady him, use your body as a slide for his body and lower both of you to the floor by sinking at your knees. (Do not lower the patient by bending your back to let him down while you remain upright: You risk severe back damage.) Flow with his fall, guiding and controlling it away from furniture or dangerous objects and using your body as a cushion to his.

6. Once the PWA is on the floor, remain with him for a while to calm his fears. When you are able, place a pillow under his head and a blanket over him until he can regain his strength to stand with you or until a friend can come to assist you in getting him back to bed. Do not attempt to lift the PWA by yourself: This can injure you as well as the patient.

The controlled fall is an important exercise to try with a friend. While you help your friend across the floor, let him "go limp"—carefully—and control his fall. Review the fall together. Did he bump anything: knees, elbows, head? How could that be avoided? Do it several more times to get the feel. It is really easier than it sounds! It's important to know how to handle a fall instinctively by having practiced it.

Personal hygiene can be especially important to an ill person. Simply having clean hair, clean teeth, and a freshly bathed body can make him feel better. After first checking with the doctor for any special precautions, file or cut fingernails and toenails. Give a male PWA the opportunity to be shaved, apply cologne, or whatever he wants to make him feel the best he can. For a woman, allow her to apply her makeup, body lotion, perfume and to paint her nails or whatever may make her feel whole.

V. **Activities of Daily Living: Personal Hygiene (Bath, Mouth Care, Skin Care)**

A. Assessment
1. Encourage the PWA to do as much for himself as possible.
2. Decide, jointly if possible, before beginning what each person will do.
3. Recognize fatigue and offer help when necessary.

B. Principles
1. *Increase Circulation.* This prevents skin breakdown. Take time to massage skin while washing, and afterward with lotion, especially over body areas and areas that appear red. Redness is a sign of skin breakdown, which leads to bedsores.
2. *Increase Muscle Tone.* Encourage the PWA to move himself around in bed and do as much of his own care as he can. This helps to maintain muscle strength and tone as well as enhance self-esteem.

C. Technique
1. *Materials Needed.* Basin (1 or 2), bedside table, soap, towels (2), washcloths (2), sheet or bath blanket, lotion, cotton swabs, powder or cornstarch, razor, toothbrush, toothpaste, gown (cover-

all), gloves. (May need Alpha Keri bath oil in water instead of soap if skin is dry.)

2. Fill basins with comfortably warm water. If skin is dry, don't use soap: Friction and warm water will clean quite well. If skin is very dry, use bath oil in the water.

3. If the PWA is able, sit him up in bed or in a chair (or in the bathtub with a nonskid mat under him) with the water, washcloths, and soap for him to wash as much of himself as possible. Offer help in hard to reach areas, such as feet and back. Keep an eye on the PWA, as he may be weak or light-headed; but be respectful of his privacy as much as possible. For instance, this may mean standing closely behind the patient if he is in a chair, ready to assist but modestly unobtrusive.

4. If giving a complete bed bath, remember again to respect modesty. Replace bedclothes and extra covers with a bath blanket, sheet, or towels. Keep the patient warm and covered at all times. Only expose and wash one part of the body at a time, such as one arm. This includes wetting, soaping, rinsing, drying, and applying lotion and powder. Use a towel under the area being washed to avoid getting bedclothes wet. If you will be coming into contact with blood, urine, feces, open sores, or other bodily fluids, wear a long-sleeved coverall and gloves.

5. Wash his face with water and cloth or cotton swabs. Move to the arm and shoulder. Soap skin, rubbing gently to increase circulation. Use the second basin for rinse water and to warm the lotion bottle. Examine each area for skin breakdown. Dry thoroughly and apply lotion and/or powder.

6. Continue bath with the other arm and shoulder, moving next to each leg and foot. Next do the

chest and finally the genital area. Complete with the back, having the PWA either sit up or roll onto his side. If he is unable to do this himself, assist him with the techniques discussed later. Follow the same routine for washing the back and buttocks. Again, check for redness and skin breakdown and finish up with a back massage.

7. While bathing, be aware of any areas that may be especially sensitive. PWAs are prone to very painful shingles (generally on the torso or head) and herpes (around the genital and rectal areas). Be aware of all sores and use the bathing time to inspect for new areas in order to report them to the medical personnel.

8. When finished, apply any medications that have been prescribed for sores and lesions. Apply powder or lotion to areas that rub together or sweat: underarms, upper thighs, genitals.

9. You may wish to wash hair by padding the bed well with towels and using one basin to catch water. Use a tearless baby shampoo. Or you may wish to use a no-rinse shampoo that doesn't require water. Discuss the options with your patient.

10. Shaving and mouth care can be done at the beginning or end of bathing, whichever the PWA prefers. If the mouth is not too sore, brush the teeth with *soft*-bristled toothbrush. Sore gums may be massaged with a clean, damp cloth or damp cotton swabs.

11. *Cleanup.* Wearing clean gloves, wash basins with soap and hot water, or run them through the dishwasher on the regular cycle. If items such as lotion bottles, powder containers, tubes of medications, and so on have been contaminated with body fluids, wash them also. If anything is noticeably contaminated with blood, wash with a 1 to 10

> bleach to water mixture. Dispose of gloves and other throwaway items in a plastic sack: Tie and toss in an outdoor garbage can.

Along with personal hygiene go clean clothing and bed linens. For a person who is spending any time at all in bed, clean, fresh sheets will be needed daily. If the PWA is incontinent (unable to control bodily functions) clothing and bed linens may have to be changed frequently during the day. If the PWA is prone to night sweats, sheets and clothing may have to be changed during the night, as well. All of this means having a extra store of bed linens available to you.

Often, clothing becomes a source of pride to a PWA when bedridden. S/he will often want to wear favorite clothes: If it makes him or her feel better, allow it. (Also, when friends want to bring gifts, clothing is appropriate: something fun, silly and comfortable, like loud-colored socks, a smoking jacket, or a crazy ball cap.) Otherwise, ordinary clothing is fine. It should be loose and comfortable and appropriately warm or cool.

VI. **Activities of Daily Living: Clothing and Bed Linens.**

    A. Assessment

        1. Watch for areas of breakdown or pressure, and protect with sheepskin or other padding as needed.

        2. If PWA is incontinent, disposable incontinence pads or diapers may have to be used. These will need to be changed as soon as possible after they have been soiled, and the PWA cleaned personally.

        3. Dress the patient according to weather, activity level, and his own comfort level. Regular clothing is fine if the PWA is up during the day. In general, clothing should be clean, not restricting or too tight, and able to be layered so that it can be easily added to or subtracted from if the PWA experiences radical changes in bodily temperature: chills, sweats, and so on.

B. Principles
   1. Clothing and bedding should be kept clean and dry.
   2. They should be changed after bathing or after bouts of incontinence or sweats.
   3. Sheepskin on elbows and heels will help prevent irritation of skin when the PWA is completely bed-ridden. Something to drape sheets over at the foot of the bed will keep pressure off feet and help prevent foot drop.
   4. When a patient is lying on his back, he may be more comfortable with pillows placed under his knees and forearms. When the patient is on his side, padding between knees and ankles and support for arms may be comfortable. In addition to sheepskin, padding may be pillows, rolled-up washcloths, folded blankets or towels.
   5. Clothing and bedding should be soft and comfortable.
   6. Tell the PWA exactly what you are going to be doing before you do it and again as you do it. This allows him to assist you as he can and doesn't scare him with the unexpected.

For a bedridden person, the condition of the bed linens can mean the difference between comfort and misery. Obviously, no one wants to lie on damp or soiled sheets. But, even when the sheets are unsoiled, they should be changed frequently. Psychologically, fresh, clean bed linens makes a patient feel fresher and cleaner.

C. Technique: Bed Linens
   1. *Materials Needed.* Fitted sheet, flat sheet, draw sheet (also called a turn sheet: a flat sheet folded in two, positioned over a fitted sheet, under patient between hips and shoulders, used in moving a PWA). Also, blankets, incontinence pads, "egg-crate" mat-

tress pad (placed between mattress and fitted sheet to prevent skin breakdown and to provide more comfort), sheepskin, pillows, other padding, and something to use at foot of bed as sheet draper for feet.

2. Bedding should be changed daily. If capable, PWA should help change linens; or, if he can't help, have him sit in a chair while bedding is being changed.

3. If the PWA is bedridden, untuck top sheets and blankets. Remove all but the top sheet for present to avoid exposing the patient. Roll the PWA onto his side near one edge of the bed (see previous instructions), making certain that all tubings (IVs, catheters, etc.) are not pulled upon or crimped. Make certain the PWA is braced so he doesn't fall out of the bed. (If a second person is available, they should hold the PWA while you make one side of the bed, then switch roles.)

4. Untuck the fitted sheet, roll the fitted sheet to the center of bed and tuck under the PWA, exposing mattress pad or egg-crate.

5. Smooth fitted sheet into place on that half of the bed. Do the same with the draw sheet and incontinence pads. Tuck excess under the PWA. There will be a lump of bedding near the center of the bed.

6. Roll the PWA over this lump onto the clean side of the bed, again bracing the PWA so he does not fall. Remove soiled linens from bed. Position fitted sheet, draw sheet, and pads. Make sure all wrinkles are smoothed out; they can cause extra pressure and lead to skin breakdown.

7. If used, place sheepskins and paddings around heels and elbows and replace drape board at foot. Remove top sheet and replace with clean top sheet and blankets.

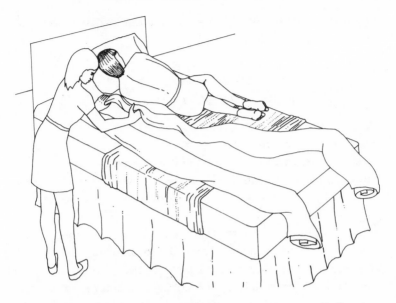

Tuck soiled sheets under patient. Start new sheets on mattress. Roll patient onto clean sheets.

Whenever possible, the PWA needs to assist himself. Simply getting out of bed has proven very beneficial for ill people. It strengthens muscles and stimulates respiration, circulation, and elimination. (Have him or her wear shoes or slippers when s/he walks so s/he doesn't bruise feet or slide.) When the patient is too weak to walk or move to a nearby chair, having the PWA sit on the edge of the bed, dangling his or her legs over the side, is also beneficial.

When a person becomes bedridden, unless s/he is alert and able to move independently, care must be taken to reposition him or her frequently (usually every two hours, and more if necessary), in order to maintain proper body alignment and prevent skin breakdown: Bedsores are almost impossible to heal and are very painful to the patient.

Lastly, the following shopping list may prove useful. Not everyone will need everything here, so pick and choose what is appropriate. It may not be necessary to buy everything: the hospital-supply houses rent equipment and some social-service agencies may have the ability to loan materials when there is an inability to pay.

walker, cane, or wheelchair

egg-crate mattress pad

extra pillows, bed sheets (fitted and flat), and blankets

a hospital bed (or a twin-sized bed raised to waist level on cement blocks) The patient needs to be where you can reach him comfortably.

extra towels and washcloths (Dark colors are preferable if there is any chance of hemorrhage: Blood on white towels looks worse than it is and causes panic in everyone.)

condom catheters or a urinal (A condom catheter is an external tube that directs urine into a urine bag, allowing a bedridden patient to relieve himself. The condoms come in different sizes.)

a bedpan and/or a porta-potty (a mobile, freestanding toilet)

underpads/incontinence pads (disposable plastic-backed pads that protect clean linen from becoming soiled)

adult diapers (to be worn under clothing if the PWA is mobile but incontinent)

two basins for bathing

a bedside table

powder (or cornstarch), lotion, bath oil for bed baths and massages

alcohol, bleach, and pine cleaner (Use a little in the mobil toilet to sanitize and kill odors.)

cotton swabs (Q-Tips)

two long-sleeved gowns or coveralls (Something you invent is less ominous looking to the PWA than surgical gowns.)

disposable face masks (to wear when *you* have a cold or cough)

disposable gloves

tearless baby shampoo or dry, no-rinse shampoo
sheepskin and small bolster pillows (especially ones with washable covers or pillow slips).

A FEW GIFT IDEAS

a wonderful, soft teddy bear or other stuffed animal (to hold on to in the middle of the night when no one is around)
a set of satin sheets (They are a luxury for the patient and make life easier on one who must slide the patient around.)
clothing: PWAs lose weight, don't fit into what they own, and can't often afford to buy new things, especially fashionable clothes. Also see introduction to Section VI., preceding, for more ideas.
gifts of service always appreciated: An offer to go grocery shopping, clean house, mow the yard, do a few loads of laundry, and so on means more to caregivers than anything you could purchase.

▪ BIBLIOGRAPHY ▪

Beland, Irene L., and Passos, Joyce Y. *Clinical Nursing: Pathopsychosocial and Psychosocial Approaches* (3rd. ed.). New York: Macmillan Publishing Co., Inc.,

Calini, Esta, R.N., Ph.D., and Owens, Gary, M.D. *Neurological and Neurosurgical Nursing* (6th. ed.). St. Louis: C.V. Mosley Co., 1974.

Ellis, Janice Rider, Nowlis, Elizabeth Ann, and Bentz, Patricia M. *Modules for Basic Nursing Skills* (2nd. ed.). Boston: Houghton-Mifflin Co., 1980.

Morbidity and Mortality Weekly Report, August 21, 1987, vol. 36, no. 25. Atlanta, Georgia: U.S. Dept. of Health and Human Services, Public Health Service, Centers for Disease Control.

15

· STORIES FROM · THE FRONT: NUMBER 4 HOW TO COPE WHEN YOUR LOVER HAS ARC OR AIDS

BILL EDWARDS

Bill Edwards is a professional in his late thirties who had been living with his lover, Art, another professional man, almost seven years at the time Art was diagnosed with *Pnuemocystis carinii* pneumonia (PCP). Within less than three months, Art developed lymphoma of the brain. The result was severe neurological damage that caused intellectual impairment and paralysis of the right side of his body. Bill drafted this chapter while on vacation with Art in the seventh month of Art's illness. Although it is written to gays who find themselves as primary caregivers to their lovers, every piece of advice in it is equally applicable to *anyone* taking care of *any person* with ARC or AIDS. What is said about looking to the gay community for support services is also valid for everyone. Though the support groups were originated within that community to help their own, they are unbiased and, in turn, are supported by many nongay volunteers. Furthermore, they will be able to refer callers to the appropriate facilities that deal with the particular concerns of drug users or other special groups.

The moment you learn your lover has ARC or AIDS, your life will begin to change. Many aspects of your new life—after that moment—will be beyond your control. But you will still determine the tenor of your life. The purpose of this chapter is to suggest ways to cope with the events that will swirl around you and the emotions that will sweep over you. To extend the metaphor, envision yourself as the captain of a ship—your life—that has entered stormy seas. Your goal is to successfully navigate the storm and emerge safely into the quiet waters that wait beyond.

The suggestions that follow are phrased briefly. Chapters or even books could be written about each of the topics covered. See the appendices at the end of the book for additional information.

▪ DEAL WITH YOUR ▪ OWN FEARS AND OTHER EMOTIONS

Your fears will be many; and fear is a normal emotion in situations such as these. It will be easy for you to imagine disasters that could result from the diagnosis of ARC/AIDS in your lover. Perhaps the worst fear—it had me in a state of panic for the first few weeks after my lover's diagnosis—is that you yourself will develop ARC or AIDS. If this fear is keeping you from coping as well as you would like, have yourself tested for infection by the HIV virus. You *may* test negative. Our doctor told us that, of lovers of ARC and AIDS patients, roughly one in five do test negative for the virus since rates of transmission vary depending on the sexual practices of the partners. If the results are positive, consider receiving counseling to help you cope with the double burden you will be bearing: your lover's present illness and the potential of your own illness. Also, since new therapies for preventing HIV-positive status from progressing to ARC or AIDS are being tested all the time, ask a knowledgeable physician what therapies may be available. You may also want to check directly with the AIDS Clinical Trials Information Service by dialing toll-free 1-800-TRIALS-A. This group will send you a free listing of all the FDA experimental HIV protocols being tested, what criteria for entry is, and where each is located.

Other fears may best be handled by reminding yourself—as often as necessary—that while some of your fears may come true, all are best dealt with when they become fact. Don't spend energy solving problems that never arise. The adage "Take one day at a time" is a good approach to this situation.

While fears should, to the extent possible, be put on hold, you will need to accept the fact that your lover could become disabled or terminally ill within a very short period of time. Do some levelheaded planning to prepare yourselves for various contingencies. See under Develop Attitudes That Will Help You Cope on page 212.

Another emotion you will certainly feel, whether you recognize it or not, is full-blown grief or just a sense of loss. This, too, is normal. When you learn that AIDS or ARC has struck your lover, you will lose many of the foundation stones of your life. Peace of mind, financial security, optimism about the future, and perhaps the love of some family and friends will all disappear. You will want to reread Chapter 12 in this book from time to time to help you cope with all of this.

Anger is yet another emotion you may have to confront. You may feel angry at your lover, yourself, the gay world, the drug culture, or other individuals or groups you see as partially or wholly responsible for your lover's illness. Acknowledge the anger—it's okay to feel it—and work toward defusing it, either through counseling or by redeveloping your own attitudes. It's not easy, but again there are some approaches listed on the following pages that I have found helpful.

• DISCUSS THE •
SITUATION WITH
YOUR LOVER

Coping must begin with good communication between yourself and your partner. All the steps suggested in the remainder of this chapter assume that you and your lover have discussed the situation and are in basic agreement on how you will face the challenges. If you have important differences of opinion that you cannot reconcile, talk to a trusted friend or a professional counselor who can help you resolve these differences.

Topics you may legitimately choose not to discuss with your lover—at least not in depth—might be your own fears, grief, or anger. Your lover will be looking to your for help in *his* or *her* dealings with these emotions. If your emotions are too strong, they may only add to his.

• DEVELOP SUPPORT •
GROUPS FOR YOUR
PARTNER AND
YOURSELF

No matter how emotionally, fiscally, and physically strong you and your partner are, you can *not* successfully cope with AIDS or ARC alone: The challenges are too many and too great. The more emotional and practical support you both have, the better you will be able to manage. Put aside any discomfort you may feel at asking others for help: You have a very legitimate need for assistance.

Before anyone can help you, they must know that ARC or AIDS is the diagnosis. Though that fact may be difficult to reveal, it should be discussed. The only possible exception may be for elderly parents or other infirm relations who simply could not cope with the knowledge. They should be told, however, that your partner is suffering from a terminal disease.

The more emotional and practical support you and your lover have while facing AIDS or ARC, the easier your coping will be. Some sources of assistance are listed here.

YOUR NETWORK OF FRIENDS. Many of your friends will want to help, but won't be sure what to do. These friends will welcome your suggestions on how they can best help you. The sort of help you need will vary, depending on your circumstances and your partner's health. Here are some ways that our friends have helped us:

> providing transportation to medical appointments
> bringing meals to the house so we didn't have to cook
> visiting in the hospital or at home during the weekdays
> doing housework and yardwork
> running errands.

LOCAL GAY ORGANIZATIONS. Most large cities have organizations that offer counseling and assistance to gay people. Many such organizations have programs specifically designed to assist ARC or AIDS patients and their loved ones. One example is the Buddy Program, which matches Persons with AIDS (PWAs) with volunteers who agree to be their buddy and assist them in a variety of ways. My lover's buddy has been a wonderful source of support and assistance for both of us; he has become one of our closest and best-loved friends. Find out what support of this type is available in your community.

MEMBERS OF YOUR FAMILY.   Many variables determine how family members react to a diagnosis of ARC or AIDS. Assuming that the families' reactions are sympathetic, you can call on them, not only for emotional support but also for the practical sorts of help discussed previously. If some family members react sympathetically and some do not, you can ask the accepting ones to help the others adjust to the situation.

PROFESSIONAL COUNSELORS.   You may wish to have a professional counselor help you cope with the emotional aspects of your situation. I visited a counselor specializing in grief, loss, and bereavement education, and she was extremely helpful to me. Another option would be to pick one or more personal friends as counselors or advisors.

RELIGIOUS ORGANIZATIONS.   A diagnosis of ARC or AIDS often leads to a revitalization of religious beliefs, even those long dormant. However, religious organizations will differ in their reaction to a diagnosis of ARC or AIDS. Some congregations and clergy—certainly those of the Metropolitan Community Churches (MCC)—will be supportive. If you and your lover have not been affiliated with a religious group but wish to join one, a local gay support organization may be able to suggest sympathetic congregations. Even if local congregations of your denomination are supportive, there also may be a gay group within your denomination to which you can turn for support. Examples are Dignity within the Roman Catholic Church, Gay Unitarians, Integrity within the Episcopal Church, Presbyterians for Gay Concerns, and Beth El Binah within the Jewish community. We were fortunate to learn of a local church sympathetic to PWAs: The outpouring of love we have received from them has kept us afloat through many turbulent times.

▪ EDUCATE YOURSELF ▪

In order to assess your situation—an important first step in coping with it—you need to know the facts about AIDS and ARC. Furthermore, many people will have questions about your lover's health, and you will need to be able to answer them authoritatively.

Many sources of information are available: your partner's physician, books and pamphlets, ARC/AIDS hotlines, and local gay support groups, just to mention some. Whatever your source, be sure your information is up-to-date; knowledge about ARC and AIDS is advancing so rapidly that materials published more than a year ago may well be out-of-date. (Refer to the appendices at the end of the book for some sources.)

As your partner's illness advances and disability sets in, you will need to educate yourself in home-nursing techniques. Ideally, you will be able to arrange for a nurse to go to your home on a regular basis. This person will be your best source of information by being able to teach you in a hands-on situation.

▪ DEVELOP ATTITUDES ▪ THAT WILL HELP YOU COPE

Probably the single most important determinant of how well you cope with your lover's illness will be the attitudes you develop about your situation. You must cultivate attitudes and thought patterns that help you cope. You will have to maintain a calm, levelheaded approach to events around you while realistically facing the situation. You cannot afford to become paralyzed by fear or grief. Examples of attitudes and thought patterns that will help you cope follow. Needless to say, talking with counselors and reading relevant materials can help you in this area.

Take one day at a time. In bad situations, the future can look overwhelmingly bleak if we envision all the problems that might face us. Focus on the problems you have to solve each day as they present themselves, and try not to worry about the problems of the future. Have a general plan for handling the future problems, but don't try to have an answer for every possibility.

Consider that each individual determines how happy s/he is in life by the way s/he views events. One fact or event, when viewed with different attitudes or perspectives, will take on different significance. Your situation will be difficult and uncomfortable, to say the least. But even in the most tragic situations, there is often much to be grateful for and happy about. For example, the expressions of love and support that we have received, often from unexpected quarters, have been a constant source of joy.

When evidence of physical decline due to the illness becomes depressing, remember these thoughts: Make no comparisons; make no judgments; delete the need to understand. That is, try not to compare present health levels with past levels. As my lover's disability progressed, I found that if I accepted the present level of health and ability, rather than comparing it with past health and ability, I was much less depressed. Often it is a matter of "letting each day define reality anew."

Remind yourself that all life is fleeting. Death is a fact of life that all of us must face sooner or later. It's how we face it, what we learn, how we love, and how we grow that's important. I recommend that you read Stephen Levine's *Who Dies?* (See Appendix F).

Remember the words "This, too, shall pass." Whatever you are experiencing—regardless how bad—is only temporary and will eventually pass away. One method I used to enforce this attitude was to envision myself at a future point in an enjoyable activity.

Despite your best efforts, you will find that your emotions fluctuate, sometimes with the moment. You may feel calm and in control one moment, and be in tears the next. Accept these mood swings as normal; have a good cry when you feel like it. Then, adjust your thought patterns to help you return to an attitude of acceptance and serenity.

▪ ACCEPT YOUR ▪ NEW ROLE AS A CAREGIVER AND MANAGER

Whatever roles you have had in your relationship until now, your lover's illness will define two new roles for you. First, you will need to assume increasing responsibility for managing your household's business and financial matters. You should be able to assume this role gradually. A first step is to be sure that your lover's will is updated. At the same time, your lover should consider completing a "Living Will" or "Directive to Physicians." This is a document that requests physicians not to take extraordinary measures to prolong life once death is near. This would also be an appropriate time to discuss his or her wishes concerning a funeral and burial. Next, you should have your lawyer draw up a document giving you Durable Power of Attorney. This document will give you authority to manage your lover's business affairs whenever s/he becomes too ill to do so. Such a document is particularly important if your lover's relatives might oppose your taking charge.

Samples of some of these forms are found in Appendix D. However, in all of this, follow the advice of your attorney. S/he will be able to lead you around the pitfalls that many stumble into: disgruntled creditors, unhappy relatives, legal responsibilities, or state inheritance laws.

A second role you will assume is that of care coordinator. You must be prepared to deal assertively with medical personnel of all levels to insure that your lover gets the best care possible. When s/he is hospitalized, you cannot assume that s/he will receive the needed attention: Be on the alert for the signs that you need to step in and act as advocate.

After hospitalization, s/he may need an attendant at home, and you may need to hire one if a friend or family member is not able to fill that role. Almost every town has a service that can supply home health aides (e.g., Visiting Nurse Association). Here also, expect that you will have to monitor performance to be sure you are both getting the help you need.

Often you will be the primary caregiver, especially on weekends and during the evenings. Be prepared for the fact that as your lover's illness advances, you will need to give progressively more care. This role may be intimidating at first, but, believe me, your comfort level will grow with practice.

▪ TAKE CARE OF ▪ YOURSELF BOTH PHYSICALLY AND EMOTIONALLY

Paradoxically, those who are caring for others often neglect to care for themselves. You must, however, take good care of yourself so you can function effectively as a caregiver. Remind yourself continually that you owe it to both yourself and your lover to eat well, get enough sleep, and find ways to manage stress. Needless to say, taking good care of yourself will become more difficult whenever your partner becomes seriously ill. So the sooner the good habits of self-care are begun, the more useful they will be.

As demands on you increase, give yourself time off from the caregiver role to relax and unwind. Get out of the house to exercise or treat yourself to a movie or dinner with friends; this will help prevent your developing "caregiver burnout." Arrange for family or friends to stay with your partner at these times; giving you time off is a favor they can do to benefit *both* you and your lover.

During your time off, consciously try not to think about your lover's illness or the problems it is causing. However, you may wish instead to contemplate the direction your life will take after your role as a caregiver is over. This is healthy and okay to do.

▪ HANG IN THERE ▪

Despite your best efforts, there will be times when you feel you simply cannot cope—with the grief, or the responsibilities, or the sheer exhaustion of constantly nursing a seriously ill person. At such times, remind yourself that "this too shall pass" and resolve to "hang in there." To return to the metaphor used in the introduction to this chapter, remember that the only way out of the storm in which you find yourself is to navigate through it as steadily as you can. You will have ups and downs as the waves toss you around, but quieter waters are awaiting you on the other side.

▪ A FINAL WORD ▪

From one who is in the midst of this as I write, I send you who read this my love and encouragement. There have been those before us; and we will make it as they have done: one day at a time.

16

·THINGS THAT· FALL THROUGH THE CRACKS

GARY SWISHER

Gary Swisher volunteered as a buddy under the Oak Lawn Counseling Center's AIDS Program in 1984. At that time, the Buddy Project was a grass-roots endeavor under the auspices of, but not supervised by, the Center. Gary was elected by the buddies themselves to be coordinator of their steering committee, a position he held until the Center hired him as its Director of Volunteer Services. Since then, he has been promoted to Director of AIDS Services, through which he coordinates the Center's AIDS services with all the other agencies. All three positions have given Gary a bird's-eye perspective of what can go wrong in any system and how the problems may best be avoided.

This chapter will attempt to address the surprise issues that may arise in the care of a PWA. As attitudes change, much of this chapter will become extremely dated material. Until then, expect to meet many challenges; expect the unexpected. Be flexible and patient. Most things can be worked out.

Whenever possible, try to plan ahead and prepare for the future. Whatever can be done before it is actually required will be greatly rewarded when crisis situations arise causing spare time and energy to be at a premium. Many of the preparations may be done relatively easily.

Begin this process by helping the PWA deal with his/her emotions. The emotional issues may seem difficult, painful, or complicated; but helping the PWA to realize, accept, and deal with newly inflicted physical, financial, and emotional limitations can lessen the difficulties.

▪ FINANCIAL MATTERS ▪

Finances are a major factor for most PWAs. Keep in mind the emotional stress involved with finances. Our society has always put a major emphasis on success. Success is measured by financial stability. Being able to pay a minimum balance due on a Visa card every month reinforces the sense of control one has over one's life.

There are several avenues for financial assistance for the general population; however, those are generally reserved for the person who can repay what is given. Attention often must be focused on indigent services and resources. Social Security is the first stopping point. Time is a critical factor with Social Security: The sooner the PWA applies, the sooner the great wheels of bureaucracy start to turn. Be advised that Social Security isn't the be-all and end-all. If someone hasn't been working or paying into the Social Security system, then there is likely nothing to receive. If Social Security isn't available or runs dry early, investigate the availability of state and local financial resources. Most areas have financial assistance for rent and utilities, at least.

No matter what sources are utilized, one point is always common: They all need pertinent (and often nonpertinent and even impertinent) information about the applicant. Experience has shown that most people do not have their personal records in neat, tidy packages. Mother may have the birth certificate. Father may have the service discharge papers. Insurance policies are with sister and past tax forms are at brother's house. Every attempt must be made to compile as complete a picture of the PWA as possible. Even if that means massive phone and letter campaigns to secure all of the important documents, it is definitely worth the effort before the PWA has to sit at an application office.

Also be advised that receiving financial assistance may not be any picnic, either. Guidelines are imposed to facilitate support services for general situations, not specific cases. AIDS has created more newly indigent people than any other disease in this century. Functioning, prosperous individuals are rapidly becoming penniless and outcast.

All too often, the restrictions placed on benefits may seem too stringent. Income and assets are limited. In more than one case, the recipient has lost benefits such as SSI (Social Security Income) and Medicaid because they were five dollars over maximum, regardless of the fact that they were not able to afford to sustain any semblance of their past life. Even glasses and/or contacts, snack foods, car payments, insurance, and so on become impossible to pay for.

▪ INSURANCE ▪

A common problem for PWAs is medical-insurance coverage. History has shown that most PWAs lose employment and, with it, their insurance coverage. However, this is not always the case. If the PWA is fortunate enough to have continued coverage, s/he may not always be aware of exactly what expenses are covered. A critical examination of all policies involved is crucial. If the PWA has several policies available, these may be able to be used in conjunction with each other to almost completely cover expenses.

Insurance companies are not the horrible monsters most of us believe them to be. They are becoming increasingly willing to negotiate policies to reduce their own expense. For example, home health care is less costly than hospitalization, and an L.P.N. or health aide may be more appropriate than an R.N. and substantially more reasonably priced. Many insurance policies may not provide for this coverage; but faced with paying the lower costs for at-home care rather than having the PWA returned to the hospital with all those costs, most companies will opt to pay for the home care.

▪ POLICIES OF ▪ ORGANIZATIONS AND THEIR MAD-HATTER SYNDROMES

In dealing with any service—federal, state, or local—organization, be very aware of their ability to change policies and procedures at a moment's notice. In past experience with a wide variety of organizations, the best results come from those that allow the PWA to deal with a single contact. The familiarity that is created reduces the fear of the unknown and unexpected for *both* parties. As with the doctor/patient relationship, building an intimacy will go a long way in procuring services from an agency.

That intimacy must go hand in hand with reliability. All too often agencies arbitrarily change policies or service provisions. These revisions are usually in response to difficult cases, overdemanding PWAs, or excessive demand on services that send agency costs skyrocketing past their budget. The most effective remedy to this type of situation has been to obtain a statement of policy when first dealing with organizations. The rule of thumb to use is, "If it is not in writing, it doesn't count." Cases have arisen where discount groceries were no longer available, dental care became more scarce, promises for reduced rents and flexible payment dates were so much wind whistling in the trees. When agreements for certain services or benefits are in writing, the agency involved will generally stand behind the promise, even after its policies change.

Guidelines from more established agencies (e.g., Social Security, Veterans Administration, etc.) are often confusing, complicated, and easy to misunderstand. How many times have you left a store, for instance, not really understanding exactly what you were agreeing to when you signed on the dotted line? Benefit agencies are no different. Though the guidelines that are established may be confusing, they are usually written to be quite specific and detailed. They must state clearly what and who qualify for benefits and what and who don't, which benefits are available and which are not. Those benefits that are not available from one agency may be supplied by another and may only require an appropriate referral. However, those referrals must be requested. More than one PWA has felt discriminated against and denied assistance because he was not informed of other support, when in reality he did not pursue further assistance of his own accord.

▪ MAINTAINING ▪ INDEPENDENCE

It is urged that the PWA try to maintain as much control in his life as possible. However, this pursuit can lead into more difficulties than bargained for. The PWA may want to keep his own home, but the result may be added expenses: mortgage or rent, utilities, plus the extra cost for sufficient physical assistance. This may add to the immeasurable stress already experienced: Where will the rent money come from? What does one do with the extra bills that there is no way of paying? How does one deal with the bill collectors who begin to harass the PWA (and maybe you, too) for payment? These become daily problems for most PWAs. Often they are not faced; rather they are avoided. The primary caregiver, whether volunteer or family member, is next in line to take over the worry and struggle to resolve the obligation. The need to take an honest look at the PWA's financial obligations and resources and the fact that a working plan must be implemented to relieve the inevitable pressure before the bill solicitors begin cannot be stressed enough.

▪ DEATH PROCEDURES: ▪ WHAT DOES YOUR AREA REQUIRE?

The scene is a typical one. The family gathers around the bedside. Someone holds the dying person's hand amidst hushed goodbyes and declared love. The eyes close, the breathing becomes shallow and then stops, the grip of the hand slackens. Tearfully, someone notifies the authorities of an expected at-home death. Now the circus begins, complete with light, sound, and action. The fire trucks come screaming down the block, sirens blaring and lights flashing. Paramedics break in and proceed to pound on the chest of the deceased and start resuscitation. Although the report had been N.R.S. (a nonresuscitation situation), the circumstances prescribed alternate measures.

What circumstances? There was no doctor or nurse present to witness the death! Also, unfortunately for this family, each area of the city (Dallas) has its own procedures for at-home death. Some areas require emergency equipment, paramedics, fire personnel, and police, regardless. Others do not.

It is strongly recommended that the county or city medical examiner's office be contacted in advance to determine precisely what procedures are to be followed. What doctor will sign the death certificate? Is there a home health agency involved? Will they supply a nurse to oversee the procedures? A great deal of stress and emotional pain may be reduced by some footwork and prearrangement. Again—"If it is not in writing, it doesn't count!"—signed letters of intent from physicians, medical examiner field agents, funeral homes, and home health care agencies can facilitate a difficult situation into a more palatable one.

The dark stages occur postmortem. In today's society, death is a taboo. It is an uncomfortable situation when viewed from any angle. Transportation and disposition of the body can result in a whole new nightmare. Be advised that if there are any signs of trauma on the body, an autopsy *must* be performed. Scars or physical damage to the body need to be noted by the physician or attending nurse *in writing* to avoid delays or suspicion of foul play.

Such was the continuing saga of the PWA mentioned above. Six years prior to his death, he was attacked and robbed. A lasting reminder was a large indentation in the side of his skull. Although the wound had healed years ago, the scars were extremely evident and were sufficient for the paramedics to demand the body be taken to the medical examiner's office for an autopsy. This unusual turn of events shocked the family and caregivers; nevertheless, they had no recourse. They were at the mercy of the public health system, which delayed transportation of the body to the funeral home, so that the funeral services had to be held in limbo.

■ FUNERAL ■ ARRANGEMENTS

Funeral services can be another sticky situation. As with any purchase, shopping around is required. Even though funeral directors' associations abound and states have set regulations on practices, not all funeral homes perform at the same level. For example, one support agency (OLCC) assisted one family in procuring services for their decreased son. Their financial sources were tapped beyond belief. The funeral home was supportive and very helpful. To ease the family's pain, services were arranged and performed gratis. Funeral homes may be willing to provide services at no charge if there are simply no financial resources or no family to fall back upon.

Not all homes are alike, though. Case in point: A family made arrangements with a local funeral home for services. During the services, guards were posted at the casket. The casket was carried by funeral home employees wearing gowns, gloves, and masks. Family and friends were required to sign releases *at* the services that released the funeral home from any liability in the event that someone contracted AIDS from being at the services!

As with any aspect of this terrible disease, fear of the unknown may cause irrational behavior on the behalf of the uneducated. Be cautious and prepared to deal with unexpected prejudice and the stigma of AIDS even from professions and individuals toward which one would normally look to receive understanding and sympathy.

Check on what services need to be performed. Is embalming required in your location? Not all states require the deceased to be embalmed. Not all states have specific restrictions on caskets. Many people are turning to the alternative of cremation. That may pose other problems. The state of Texas requires all living relatives to sign a release and agreement to have the body cremated. If one of the relatives refuses, the cremation cannot take place. Are there restrictions in the disposal of the ashes after cremation? Wishes of scattering ashes cover seas or geographic areas may be romantic; however, the reality may be more harsh given local restrictions.

■ WILLS ■

When the funeral is over, the survivors may have to carry on with more uncomfortable business. First, the disposition of belongings is not an easy matter. Wills are undeniably one of the best planning tools and should always be utilized. Several cases have become even more painful as family and friends began to battle over belongings. Although AIDS is a health issue rather than a moral one, the relationship of survivors can become a hornet's nest. If a lover or significant other is to be left as beneficiary, s/he has no recourse or claim to the belongings of the person s/he may have spent a larger part of life with unless it is specifically provided for in a will. Family members have been known to vent their anger and pain for their child's demise at his or her surviving lover. In some cases, parents have stripped homes bare of all possessions. Siblings have cleaned out bank accounts. Family members have locked surviving partners out of their own homes and removed vehicles. Even nonrelated friends have become the proverbial "vultures" and laid claim to belongings that may or may not have been promised by the deceased prior to his or her death. As always, "If it is not in writing, it doesn't count."

What of the PWA who dies totally indigent: Is a will necessary? You better believe it! Although there may not be any belongings to disseminate, personal wishes regarding funeral arrangements may be carried out specifically because the time was taken to have a legal document written enforcing what was desired.

▪ CONCLUSION ▪

These are but a few of the events that may occur. For those who take every opportunity to plan in advance for the crises that occur in 30 percent of AIDS cases, such happenings are able to be taken in stride, being neither very surprising nor painful. However, for the unwary and unprepared, they can be devastating. Remember to document everything! And if it seems appropriate, make copies and pass them out like advertising flyers to all concerned. A majority of the problems and surprises people have faced can be alleviated by coordination, communication, and commitment.

If you need help to get everything together or to discuss delicate matters with the PWA, get it! But, do it now! Don't let it fall through the cracks.

·SECTION IV·

INDIVIDUAL POPULATIONS

17

· THE HIV-INFECTED · CHILD

MARY MALLORY, R.N.C., P.N.P., AND LYDIA ALLEN, R.N., B.S.N.

Mary Mallory and Lydia Allen work with HIV-infected children at Children's Medical Center in Dallas, Texas. Mary is the ARMS (AIDS-Related Medical Services) Clinic Coordinator and Pediatric Nurse Practitioner. Previously, she worked with HIV-infected children through Bryan's House (an HIV children's day-care center) in Dallas. Lydia is the Educational Support Nurse for the Bureau of Maternal Child Health–funded Pediatric HIV Demonstration Project and has been involved with children with HIV since 1982.

For more than a decade, people have been dealing with HIV-infected children—silently, behind the closed doors of homes and hospitals. In most cases, the children weren't seen. Some were hidden or even abandoned in hospitals. Others were locked in almost sterile rooms in overprotective homes. Over the past few years, as HIV-infected children have emerged into the public view, and as hospitals and agencies have become more used to dealing with the special problems of these children on a routine basis, a middle course of child care has emerged.

Today, care of an HIV-infected child of any age is more balanced between conscientious observation and normal social integration. In other words, parents and caregivers are asked to make the child's life as normal and rewarding as possible, to raise the child with as much love and attention as they would any child, and to allow the child to get into the same kinds of scrapes other children get into. At the same time, parents and caregivers are asked to be attentive to developmental growth, physical changes, and the appearance of rashes, ailments, fevers, et cetera.

It is not an easy balance to strike. On the one hand, you are being told, "Don't be overprotective"; but on the other hand, you're told, "Be cautious." Before becoming too frustrated, though, just remember that parents and guardians of perfectly healthy children have been given the same mixed messages for years!

This chapter will give you the steps you can take in maintaining a normal home environment and will also present the warning signals that mandate caution. It may feel awkward at first, but have faith: You *will* find the balance and it *will* become part of your routine.

• DUAL-CARE ISSUES •

Taking care of an HIV-infected child is seldom done in a vacuum. Parents may have other children and possibly brothers, sisters, or elderly relatives who also require attention. Caregivers may have spouses and other people who are equally important in their lives and who also need and expect love and care. As well, the parent/caregiver of an infected child is often HIV-positive him- or herself, and may require medical attention and support as much as if not more than the child in order to be there for the child when needed.

All these calls for attention, love, and care are valid. Each is equally important. Caring for an HIV-infected child must be balanced with caring for the rest of the family and for yourself. Other chapters in this book will be helpful in helping you recognize and meet other family members' needs as well as your own. If you are an infected mother, you will want to read the chapter relating to women and AIDS. If you are the spouse of an infected adult, you will want to read the earlier chapters on psychosocial issues and grief.

Remember that as the parent/caregiver of an HIV-infected child, the goal is to strike a balance. You will have to make many of your decisions through guesswork and informed hunches. In retrospect, many decisions may seem wrong. There are few rights and wrongs in the management of HIV disease, for it is still largely an unknown field. Parents and caregivers will almost always do the best they can under the circumstances: Be Easy on Yourself!

▪ NATURAL HISTORY ▪

Though HIV disease affects the black and Hispanic populations residing in lower socioeconomic areas at a higher rate than it does other groups, the disease knows no boundaries. Women of every age, race, and socioeconomic class can become infected and transmit the virus to their children. However, there have been no known cases of transmission from child to child, even in the same household.

The majority of perinatal transmissions occur in IV-drug-using mothers. Women may also become infected sexually from an infected partner or from contaminated blood products. (See Chapter 1.)

Some children acquire the infection from a blood transfusion, but most acquire it from an infected mother during pregnancy or delivery. A woman can carry the virus and transmit it to her unborn child without ever having symptoms of the disease. Frequently, a woman may go undiagnosed until her child becomes ill.

- Currently, about 20 to 30 percent of babies born to HIV-positive mothers are themselves infected.
- The majority of these children will be diagnosed by their second birthday; with the new PCR (Polymerase Chain Reaction) tests, the diagnosis may be made within the first two months of life.
- The child may be the first family member identified as being infected. This will require screening of parents and siblings for the virus and the provision of appropriate education and counseling.
- Early recognition is important to ensure appropriate instructions for home care and regular medical follow-up. Early treatment is beneficial in delaying the onset of HIV symptoms and illness.
- Opportunistic infections in the first year are associated with higher mortality.
- The most common opportunistic infections are pneumocystis carinii pneumonia (PCP), a pneumonia that only people with poor immune function get, and candida esophagitis (thrush in the throat).
- Failure to thrive and poor weight gain are persistent complaints.
- Lymphadenopathy (swollen lymph glands), hepatosplenomegaly (enlarged liver and spleen), and persistent oral thrush (white patches in the mouth that don't rub off) are common symptoms.
- Tumors (cancers) can occur but are very rare in children.
- It is common for children with AIDS to be anemic (low red blood counts) and to have elevated liver enzymes (blood tests indicating how the liver functions) and elevated immunoglobulins (blood tests showing how the immune system functions).

▪ Neurological symptoms in children include the failure to achieve developmental milestones or the loss of developmental milestones.

▪ TESTING ▪

Testing of children born to HIV-infected mothers is not usually done until the child is six to nine months old. The tests used are the same antibody tests used for adults: the ELISA and the Western Blot. Because the mother's antibodies are present in the baby, the tests may show positive antibody results for the first fifteen to eighteen months even if the child is not infected. Current tests do not discriminate between mother's antibody and baby's antibody; therefore, babies born to HIV-infected mothers will test positive for an average of fifteen months. As the mother's antibody diminishes in the baby, the tests may be indeterminate before turning negative. Repeated testing every three months is a common practice until a definite diagnosis is made, or until the child has two negative antibody tests. A baby that ultimately tests negative has always been negative and healthy, and will remain so. A child who tests positive at eighteen months is considered HIV-infected.

The PCR (Polymerase Chain Reaction) is a newer test. It looks at the virus in the body instead of at the antibody (the body's defense system) *to* the virus. At this time, the test is expensive, performed in only a few cities, and still being studied to determine its accuracy. If it proves to be effective, doctors will be able to diagnose babies much earlier than at present.

HIV testing requires signed informed consent by the patient, parent, or legal guardian. Laws concerning confidentiality of test results vary from state to state. You may get the most up-to-date information on the law and the location of testing sites by calling your local health department. Testing should also be available at your local children's hospital or medical center. It is also widely available through Planned Parenthood associations and prenatal-care clinics.

▪ MAKING TREATMENT ▪ DECISIONS

In choosing your physician, you will want one who either knows about childhood HIV or will be in close touch with an HIV specialist. You will want a doctor with whom you feel comfortable asking questions and whose answers you understand.

Making treatment decisions for an HIV child is difficult. Many of the treatments are preventive, that is, to keep an infection from occurring. In making any treatment decision it may be helpful to:

1. Talk with other parents of HIV-infected children.
2. Read articles about the treatment in question.
3. Try to assess what the impact on the whole family will be over a period of time: Does the treatment require travel? How often? What will the cost be? What is the time commitment? What is the physical cost (many experimental drugs require extra blood drawings or other monitoring)?
4. Ask what the expected outcome will be—with and without treatment.
5. Ask about alternatives.
6. Remember that while you have the right to refuse any test or treatment you consider unnecessary or excessive, it is best to get a second opinion before doing so.

Some caregivers make these decisions by asking themselves, "Will this improve the quality of my child's life? Or will getting this treatment be so disruptive that it takes away quality?" For instance, one family decided that once-a-month I.V.'s at the local hospital were acceptable but that traveling cross-country once every few weeks to an experimental drug study would be too disruptive and draining. If there are siblings involved, their care and emotional well-being must also be considered when making long-term decisions.

▪ IMMUNIZATIONS ▪

In order to prevent what could be life-threatening diseases, HIV-positive and HIV-indeterminate children should be immunized as long as their overall health allows. Routine vaccinations for diphtheria, pertussis, tetanus (DPT) and polio are given (a killed form of polio [IPV] is used instead of the oral [OPV]). The MMR (measles/mumps/rubella) vaccine can be given as regularly scheduled.

Your child's pediatrician should be notified immediately if your child is exposed to chicken pox. Your child may receive VZIG (varicella zoster immune globulin), which is an injection of immunoglobulin against varicella zoster, the virus causing chicken pox. The VZIG seems to lessen the severity of the outbreak if it occurs. Some HIV-infected adults have experienced shingles after exposure to chicken pox and therefore need to notify their own physician of an exposure. Exposure to Fifth's disease is also a reason to notify your physician. Fifth's disease can cause a drop in total red blood cells that can be severe, and the physician will want to watch for this. Intravenous gamma globulin (IVGG) for three consecutive days may correct this problem.

▪ ANTIVIRAL THERAPY ▪

AZT (zidovudine) Retrovir is now FDA-approved for children's use and is available through your physician. Children have fewer side effects from it than adults do but can develop anemia, headaches, and nausea. Some physicians suggest starting a child's AZT treatment with a small dose and then increasing a little every few days until reaching the correct amount. Giving AZT with meals or snacks may decrease the headaches and nausea. Keeping light snacks—crackers and fruit—in the stomach throughout the day and at bedtime also seems to decrease the nausea. After the initial adjustment to AZT, these side effects cease.

AZT must be given in divided doses on a regular basis for life or until other treatments are available. It *must* be continued even though your child looks and feels good. The virus will start reproducing when the AZT levels drop. Consult your local health department for the availability of state assistance programs for AZT in your area.

ddI and ddC are newer drugs now being studied at research sites across the country. They are available to children enrolled in these drug studies. For more information on new investigational drugs, contact the National Institute of Health in Bethesda, Maryland: 1-800-TRIALS-A.

■ PHYSICAL PROBLEMS OF ■
HIV INFECTION

HIV infection usually follows a chronic disease pattern. This means that there will be episodes of deterioration and illness followed by periods of well-being. Most HIV-infected children will have various symptoms over the course of their illness, including failure to thrive (that is, not growing), recurring thrush, anemia, breathing difficulty, fevers, skin rashes, and chronic diarrhea.

Common effects of HIV infection are discussed below. As a parent/caregiver, you will recognize changes in your child's activity level, appetite, and mood that indicate when he/she is not feeling well. Sometimes it is difficult to know if the symptoms are normal childhood illnesses, HIV related, or the result of an opportunistic infection. It is important to report these changes in your child's condition to your pediatrician, especially if fever is present. Early medical intervention can lessen or avert many illnesses and help maintain your child's strength.

• MEDICAL PROBLEMS •

• SWOLLEN GLANDS • (LYMPHADENOPATHY)

Many children experience swollen lymph nodes during illness, and some nodes will remain swollen for long periods even when your child doesn't appear ill. These nodes can be in the neck, groin, or under the arm. There is no medicine to reduce the swelling, although regular intravenous gamma globulin (IVGG) seems to alleviate this problem in some children. IVGG (harvested antibodies acquired from blood donations) works for the immune system the same way that a blood transfusion works for the blood system. This extra protection lasts only a few weeks and therefore is repeated periodically.

• RESPIRATORY DIFFICULTIES •

Many children with HIV infection will breathe faster than usual, cough frequently, and have respiratory infections that may require a hospital stay. PCP (pneumocystis carinii pneumonia) and LIP (lymphoid interstitial pneumonia) are types of respiratory problems your child may develop. If your child has difficulty breathing, it may be helpful to elevate the head of the bed or place the child in a sitting position. Report any breathing problems or color changes to your pediatrician.

• FEVERS •

A temperature under the arm above 101 degrees Fahrenheit is a sign of infection. If your child's temperature stays this high longer than twenty-four hours, notify your pediatrician. HIV-infected children frequently have fevers for days or even weeks at a time. Your doctor may suggest a fever reliever to help control the fever and make your child more comfortable. You will be given instructions on how much and how frequently to give this medicine. If your child is on AZT, do not use acetaminophen (Tylenol). Instead, use aspirin or ibuprofen.

▪ RASHES AND SORES OF THE SKIN ▪

Rashes and sores are common and can be a sign of infection. Notify your pediatrician if one appears. Rashes may also occur as a side effect of medication or an allergy. Intact skin is the first line of defense against germs and other harmful organisms. It is important to bathe your child daily, dry him/her well, and use lotions to prevent too-dry skin and irritation.

▪ DEVELOPMENTAL DELAY ▪

Neurological complications are sometimes the first sign of illness in children with congenital HIV infection. These neurodevelopmental abnormalities are often so extensive and debilitating that they can be the most difficult and frustrating aspect of HIV infection in children. Typical abnormalities include developmental delay, loss of developmental milestones, microcephaly (abnormal smallness of the head), and cognitive defects. These problems develop as a result of HIV directly infecting various structures of the brain. Some HIV-infected children will experience a slow, progressive deterioration of their mental capabilities, including failure to attain new developmental milestones or developing at a slower rate. Early developmental and cognitive testing can be helpful in ascertaining proper educational placement and selection of services.

Children on antiviral therapy—AZT, ddI or ddC—have improved developmentally, and it is now thought that much developmental delay can be avoided by early intervention with antivirals.

▪ FAILURE TO THRIVE ▪

Many children with HIV infection have problems gaining weight and growing as fast as others their age. The cause of this is not always known but may be due to HIV or another infection. It can also be caused by poor appetite, vomiting, and diarrhea. Antiviral therapies have helped many children start to grow, gain appetites, and decrease vomiting and diarrhea. A nutritionist can help you with diet plans and ways to increase calorie intake for your child.

▪ OPPORTUNISTIC INFECTIONS ▪ (REFER TO AIDS CHART TWO)

▪ BACTERIAL AND VIRAL INFECTIONS ▪

Children with HIV may experience a greater number of ear, sinus, and upper-respiratory infections. Your pediatrician may be aggressive in treating these, especially those accompanied by high fevers. Intravenous gamma globulin (IVGG) has been used since 1981 to reduce the incidence of bacterial infections. This is given one to two times a month on an outpatient basis. The need for regular IVGG is determined by the number of infections a child has, his/her ability to overcome the infection, and weight and growth factors.

▪ PNEUMOCYSTIS CARINII ▪ PNEUMONIA (PCP)

PCP is an organism that infects the lungs, causing severe pneumonia. Symptoms include fever, cough, rapid breathing, and fatigue. The child may be placed on trimethoprim/sulfa (marketed as oral Bactrim or Septra) to prevent the infection from developing. Children have very few side effects from this drug. Bactrim/Septra has been shown to be effective when used continually three days a week. It is the drug of choice due to its low cost and the fact that it is easy to take. It is very important that this medicine be given for the duration of the child's life. Aerosolized pentamidine has been used in children as young as six years old who are intolerant to Bactrim/Septra. The child must be compliant and able to follow instructions for proper use of the nebulizer (a machine that turns the liquid medicine into a breathable mist).

▪ CANDIDA (THRUSH) ▪

Although thrush is a normal, treatable occurrence in many babies, it is difficult to control in children with AIDS. This fungus can occur in the mouth or the esophagus, or on the skin in the diaper area. Candida on the inside of the mouth looks like curdled milk and can make eating and drinking painful. Drugs used to control this fungus are Mycostatin, Mycelex Troche, and Nizoral Liquid. A new drug, fluconazole, is an oral (pill) antifungal medication that is very effective in controlling thrush.

▪ HERPES ▪

Herpes is a virus causing lesions in the mouth, making it painful to eat or drink. Acyclovir (Zovirax) is prescribed in cream or pill form, or intravenously if the child is hospitalized.

▪ GIVING MEDICATIONS ▪

Children can be taught to take pills at a very early age, which will lessen your medication-preparation time. Try giving a pill in a spoonful of yogurt, jelly, pudding, or applesauce. Often, children will be on several oral medications: It is very important that they be given according to schedule. Do not use medications as punishment or threats. Initially when teaching the child to take medication, be firm, and then offer a small treat when he/she has finished. Soon the treat will not be needed. Do not belittle the child by saying that the medicine "could not be that bad." Acknowledge that you know it tastes bad and that you understand that the child doesn't want to take it, but that there are *no options.* The child may be given the option as to what food or drink will be taken with the medication.

■ SOCIALIZATION ■

It is oversimplistic (but nonetheless true) to say that HIV affects the whole family, not just the individuals infected. Before telling people outside the immediate family, it may be wise to allow the shock of the diagnosis to lessen *within* the family. This usually takes three to six months' time. The family/caregivers then have time to plan a strategy that will be the most helpful to the adults, the HIV-infected child, and other children in the family, if any. It is important to remember that even though other family members may not be infected with HIV, they may be affected socially as if they were. Choose carefully whom you tell.

Before taking anyone into your confidence, consider the following:

1. Does this person *need* to know?
2. Do *you* need this person to know for *your* own support? Is this person able to give you that support? How much does this person know about HIV?
3. What might this person's reaction be?
4. Are you prepared for rejection if the person is unable to accept the HIV-infected child?
5. If the reaction is negative, will it affect
   a. anyone's employment or livelihood? (One family chose to be very private because they sold produce

          locally and were concerned that their customers
          might be afraid to purchase their vegetables.)

  b. the family's housing situation?

  c. older children's friends or school experiences?

  d. church membership or attendance (the child's admittance into church day care, for instance)?

Federal law (P.L.-94-142) protects the rights of children to a free and appropriate public education if they have a disability and a need for special education and related services. Both the U.S. Public Health Service and the Centers for Disease Control strongly recommend that all HIV-infected children be included in the regular public-education system. Many states require that only those who "need to know," such as the school nurse, are to be told about a child's HIV status. In some states, the child's condition need not be revealed at all; even the school nurse is not informed. Caregivers should check with their local school district for information concerning confidentiality.

▪ COPING WITH A ▪ CHRONICALLY ILL CHILD

As you care for your chronically ill child, your physical and emotional energies may often be drained. For you to be able to "go the distance," you must care for yourself. (See Chapter 10 on stress and burnout.)

Even if you have the support of extended family or friends, it may still be helpful for you to turn to community agencies. Some areas of the country have day and/or respite (overnight) care for HIV-infected children. Others provide home-attendant help. Often, there are parent-support groups where caregivers can talk about stress, medical-care concerns, and medical advances; at the very least, such groups will help you feel less lonely and alone. See what is available in your area to help you. A hospital social worker may have the names of such organizations; your local health department is also a good referral source.

Find a few other warm hands and bodies, and allow them to get to know your child. This will help you to gain trust in those individuals and to share the physical care of the child when you need assistance. Child care is demanding in the best of circumstances; with the added stress of HIV, getting "breaks" is paramount, and having a special "aunt" or "uncle" visit becomes a treat. You need the time to replenish your reserves. Your time off benefits everyone, especially the ill child. This is particularly true if you also are HIV-positive and need to conserve your own health!

In summary:

1. Recruit extra hands.
2. Get away regularly, even if it is only to the backyard or to a movie.
3. Talk to other parents.
4. Get in touch with community agencies that offer assistance, and take advantage of what is available to you and your child.

▪ ASSISTING THE CHILD ▪ TO COPE

Whether or not you choose to use the terms "HIV," "ARC," or "AIDS" with your child, the child will sense that he/she is not like others, that he/she is somehow different. Children read faces, voices, and moods. They are extremely intuitive. That is why limited honesty can be useful. "Limited honesty" means answering truthfully questions directly asked by the child and saying *no more* ("Why do I have to take medicine?" . . . "You need this medicine to help you stay healthy" . . . "Bobby doesn't have to take medicine, why do I?" . . . "Bobby doesn't need it, his body works differently; like blue eyes and brown eyes, everyone is different.").

It is important that all the adults involved with the child talk about and agree upon a terminology to be used, in order to avoid confusing the child. If confidentiality is a major concern, you may wish to keep explanations simple. It may be too great a burden for a young child not to tell everything he/she knows to playmates, the supermarket checker, or neighbors.

When it is necessary for the child to have lab tests or treatments, remember that you may be in for a long ordeal. Try to make the experience as pleasant as possible while acknowledging how difficult it may be for the child. This will pay off in future medical visits. Avoid sermonizing, harsh tones, and severe punishments. It is perfectly understandable that the child does not want to cooperate and protests what is being done to him/her. Obstinacy at this point does not fall into the same category as not picking up one's toys.

At treatment time it may be helpful to:

1. Explain the treatment, taking into account the child's age and maturity.
2. Follow the child's lead in giving information.
3. Allow the child to make as many decisions as possible —this decreases his/her fear (for example: "Do you want to sit up or lie down?"). Caution: Do not give the child options if there really aren't any—this will lead to distrust in the future.
4. Assist the child to deal with his/her anticipation of pain by:
   a. Diverting with stories, games, or toys during setup.
   b. Telling the child immediately before a painful event occurs, but not long enough before to build up anxiety.

c. Being honest about what's involved (for example: "This may sting; now, close your eyes and squeeze my hand").

d. Diverting again immediately after ("That must have hurt—let's play a game that's fun").

e. Later, encourage the child to talk about his/her hurt, anger, et cetera.

f. Allow the child to perform the pain-causing act on a doll or toy.

Some parents prefer not to be present during unpleasant medical procedures, but to be the "rescuer" once the unpleasantness is over. This is a normal reaction and perfectly acceptable.

A favorite toy may be of comfort during procedures that hurt. Allowing a child to dress up as a fantasy character may also help him/her to escape mentally ("I'm not Bobby, I'm Batman!"). The costume need not be elaborate, since the child's imagination is in play: A towel and a safety pin for a cape may suffice. The child's dressing up also gives medical personnel a way to relate to him/her in a nonthreatening and fun manner, which helps to reduce the child's anxiety.

Some suggestions for helping your child to cope:

1. Enjoy your child: Try to have some fun every day. Many children have only minor problems for years.

2. Have all the adults significantly involved with the child agree on the information and the terminology to be used (for example: "You have a blood problem" or "You have a disease caused by a virus").

3. Children have a limited sense of the future: Take your cues from the child and focus on *now*.

4. Allow the child to talk about "when I grow up." This may be very difficult for you. Try to focus on, say, a

career: "Oh, you are interested in fire fighters? Let's visit the fire station."

5. Allow the child to take the lead in questions about health and illness at his or her level of readiness. Give answers the same way you would give reproductive information: a little at a time. Give only the information asked for, and as briefly as possible. If the child wants more, he/she will ask.

6. Reflect for the child what he is experiencing: "It's no fun to get all the needles; I'd be mad too!"; "You don't have to like the medicine, but you do have to take it."

▪ A WORD OF CAUTION ▪

Although home life needs little change to accommodate someone with HIV, there are a few precautions that should be taken. Normal dish washing and laundry procedures are sufficient. For a child in diapers, thorough hand washing after the change is a must. Gloves must be worn by anyone assisting the child with stools, blood, or vomit. Disposable diapers are recommended, both for their convenience and to lessen contact with urine and stool. Disposables may be discarded in regular plastic trash bags. Cleanliness is a good common practice, but remember that most of the infections affecting persons with HIV are caused by factors from within the person, not from the environment. Also, the HIV-related ailments a child might have *are not contagious to others in the family.*

When other children in the family have colds, et cetera, it is extremely difficult for caregivers to prevent the HIV-infected child from catching them. Overprotection and isolation are more detrimental than helpful. Remember that *all* children have colds and flus; the HIV-infected child will have his/her share as well.

▪ BASIC GUIDELINES FOR FOODS ▪

1. All meats should be well cooked.
2. When handling raw meat in food preparation, wash your hands before touching other utensils or you may put harmful bacteria into other foods.
3. Plastic cutting boards should be used for cutting meats—wooden ones allow bacteria to grow.
4. Raw eggs (as in Caesar salads, for instance) and meats and unpasteurized cheeses are a high risk for people with immune problems.
5. In foreign travels: Boil it, peel it, bake it, or avoid it. Use only sterilized water.

▪ PETS ▪

Caregivers may be concerned that pets may unduly expose a child to infections he/she would not otherwise come in contact with. With normal cleanliness and veterinary care (shots, et cetera), pets should not be a problem. Dogs and cats cannot acquire HIV from an infected child, even if the animal nips and bites. If a child is bitten, the wound should be cleaned thoroughly and your doctor should be called for instructions.

Precautions concerning pets:

1. Children should not be allowed to walk barefoot where there are dog or cat droppings.
2. Cat litter should be changed often and regularly—ideally by an HIV-negative person. If the changer has HIV, the litter should be covered and gloves should be worn.
3. It is recommended that birds not be kept in HIV households, as they may expose immune-compromised people to mycobacterium avium intracellare (an infection similar to tuberculosis), which is very difficult to treat.

COMPLICATIONS OF HIV INFECTION IN CHILDREN

Disease	Treatment
I. Opportunistic Infections:	
pneumocystis carinii pneumonia (PCP)	trimethoprim-sulfa methoxazole (TMP-SMX), pentamidine
Candida thrush *Candida* esophagitis	Nystatin, clotrimazole troches (Mycelex), ketoconazole
cytomegalovirus (CMV)	ganciclovir (Cytovene), foscarnate (Foscavir)
mycobacterium avium (MAI or MAC)	none completely effective, but have included ansamycin, clofazimind, ethambutol, amikacin, isoniazid, etionamide, and clarithromycin
cryptosporidiosis	no effective therapy
cryptococcus	amphotericin B, 5-flucytocine, or fluconazole (Diflucan)

Diagnosis made by open-lung biopsy or bronchoalveolar lavage. Poor prognosis if occurs before 12 months. Prophylaxis 3 days/wk. indicated for children born to HIV-infected mothers with CD4 counts below normals for age. (See *MMWR* 1991 40:1-13.) Symptoms include fevers, rapid respiration, fatigue.

White patches in mouth (thrush) or esophagus. Oral Nystatin used as initial treatment but may require additional treatments. Mycelex troches work well when crushed and mixed with small amounts of water to make paste. Paste can be rubbed over oral lesions. Appetite may decrease during periods with thrush. Relapses common and may require maintenance therapy.

Although common in the general population, may result in problems for the immunocompromised child. Can cause chorioretinitis, pneumonitis, hepatitis, colitis, esophagitis, and encephalitis. HIV-infected infants who are CMV-antibody-negative should receive only CMV-negative blood.

Disseminated infection (blood, bone marrow, liver, spleen, GI tract). Most common presentation in children is GI with pain, bloating, and diarrhea.

May cause a gastroenteritis that can lead to malnutrition. Chronic infection.

May cause meningitis, fungemia, or pneumonia. After initial daily treatment for 4–6 weeks, lifelong weekly treatment with amphotericin B or Fluconazole is given.

Disease	Treatment
II. Other Infections:	
herpes simplex	acyclovir (Zovirax): orally, I.V., and topical.
varicella zoster	acyclovir
salmonella	trimethoprim-sulfa (TMP-SMX)
respiratory infections, e.g., rhinitis, otitis media, sinutitis, pneumonia.	10-14–day course with usual antibiotics. Intravenous immune globulin (IVIG)
Post–exposure to measles	IVIG
Post–exposure to varicella	Varicella Zoster Immune Globulin (VZIG)
III. Lymphocytic Interstitial Pneumonia (LIP):	
	long-term oxygen, steroids

Recurrences frequent and may require ongoing therapy. May cause lesions on the mouth and lips. This can cause difficulty in feeding. Cool beverages are usually tolerated well.

Chronic or relapsing lesions usually occur around the waist or down the legs. Lesions can be painful and may require medication. Indications for and effectiveness of oral therapy are not clear. Mild cases may respond to oral acyclovir.

Recurrent episodes may warrant prolonged courses of antibiotics.

I.V. vs. oral therapy depends on clinical severity. Recurrent infections are common. Cram-negative pathogens (pseudomonas/klevsiella) require IV antibiotics. I.V.IG has been proven useful in children in decreasing the incidence of infections requiring hospitalizations.

Measles vaccine indicated on regular immunization schedule.

Will not prevent an outbreak of chicken pox but will lessen the severity. Must be given as soon as possible after exposure, within 96 hours.

Chronic condition unique to children. Exact cause unknown. May be progressive and lead to chronic oxygen dependence.

Disease	Treatment
IV. Other Organ Systems:	
cardiac	management of arrhythmias and congestive heart failure from myocardiopathy
renal	maintenance of fluid and electrolyte balance
liver	no effective therapy
bone marrow anemia	blood transfusions to keep hemoglobin (Hgb) over 8 gms
thrombocytopenia	IVIG
V. Chronic Pain:	
	Tylenol and ibuprofen may be helpful at first; oral, intravenous, and intramuscular narcotics may be indicated

Comments

Muscle dysfunction often poorly responsive to therapy.

Other causes of liver disease should be sought.

EPO may be tried if anemia due to decreased erothropoietin levels.

May be autoimmune process.

Headache and abdominal pain are the most common. Pain is often over-looked in children; caregivers can be very helpful in identifying if the child is in pain.

▪ **RESOURCES** ▪

National Pediatric HIV Resource Center
Children's Hospital of New Jersey
15 South Ninth Street
Newark, New Jersey 07107
(201) 268-8251

Association for the Care of Children's Health
3615 Wisconsin Avenue N.W.
Washington, D.C. 20016
(202) 244-1801

Children's Hospice International
1101 King Street, Suite 131
Alexandria, Virginia 22314
(703) 684-0330
1-800-2-4-CHILD

National Institutes of Health
Building 10
9000 Rockville Pike
Bethesda, Maryland 20892

National Information Center for Children and Youths with
    Handicaps
P.O. Box 1492
Washington, D.C. 20013
1-800-999-5599

The ARC (The Association for Retarded Citizens of the
    United States)
P.O. Box 1047
Arlington, Texas 76004
1-800-433-5255

▪ BIBLIOGRAPHY ▪

American Academy of Pediatrics, Task Force on Pediatric AIDS. "Pediatric Guidelines for Infection Control of Human Immunodeficiency Virus (Acquired Immunodeficiency Virus) in Hospitals, Medical Offices, Schools and Other Settings." *Pediatrics,* Vol. 82, No. 5, Nov. 1988.

Boland, Mary, and Deborah Rizzi. *The Child With AIDS: A Guide for the Family.* Newark: United Hospitals Medical Center, 1986.

Durham, Jerry, and Ferissa Cohen. *The Person with AIDS—Nursing Perspectives,* 2nd ed. New York: Springer Publishing Co., 1991.

Frantz, Thomas T. *When Your Child Has a Life-Threatening Illness.* Washington, D.C.: Association for the Care of Children's Health, 3615 Wisconsin Avenue N.W., Washington, D.C. 20016 ($5.50, including shipping), 1983.

McCarroll, Tolbert. *Morning Glory Babies.* New York: St. Martin's Press, 1988.

National Association of State Boards of Education. "Someone at School Has AIDS." 1012 Cameron Street, Alexandria, Virginia 22314 ($5.00 prepaid).

RN-AIDSLINE. Vol. 3, No. 3, Summer 1991. Table 3, p. 3.

Scott, Gwendolyn B. "Clinical Manifestations of HIV Infection in Children." *Pediatric Annals,* May 1988.

Swain, Jonathan, and Sharon Schilling. *My Name Is Jonathan (and I Have AIDS).* Denver: Prickly Publishing and Consulting Co., 1989.

Wiznia, A., and A. Rubinstein. "Acquired Immunodeficiency Syndrome in Infants and Children." *Annales Nestle,* Vol. 46, 1988.

18

·ALCOHOL AND· DRUG ABUSE AND AIDS

JUDY K. LOCKE, M.A., M.DIV.

Judy Locke is a Texas Certified Drug and Alcohol-ism Counselor and a staff member at Parkside Lodge-Westgate in Denton, Texas, a treatment center and hospital. She is the cofounder and facilitator of Positive AIDS in Recovery (PAR), a Twelve Step support group for recovering alcohol-ics and addicts who are HIV-positive.

The effect of alcohol and drug abuse on health and behavior is an important issue in the treatment of HIV infection. It is also a significant issue for caregivers and service providers who work and care for HIV-infected individuals.

When drug and alcohol use begins to affect the health or behavior of persons with AIDS-Related Complex (ARC) or AIDS, then their use is no longer a matter of personal, private consequence. Both those who are HIV infected and their care-givers feel the impact.

The purpose of this chapter is to discuss the drug and alcohol issues associated with AIDS and to offer those of you who are caregivers some specific suggestions for coping and helping.

Of course, AIDS is not the only disease that can be complicated or intensified by alcohol and drugs. But because alcohol and drugs can cause adverse changes in the immune system, their use can cause rapid decline in the health of persons who are HIV infected. In addition, the behavior of persons under the influence can put a strain on relationships and create additional challenges for their caregivers. Finally, community agencies and service providers may limit the help they offer to HIV-infected persons with histories of drug and alcohol abuse or whose chemical use affects their ability to cooperate and to share resources. As community resources and services are precious enough, individuals' drug or alcohol use and/or their resulting behavior may determine the availability of services and, in some cases, may require abstinence and sobriety. This creates even more problems for the caregivers.

This chapter is designed to help you recognize and identify drug and alcohol *abuse,* understand why abuse is truly a problem, and direct you toward the proper resources.

• ALCOHOL AND DRUG USE • AND HEALTH

The seriousness of the effect of alcohol and drug use on a person's health depends on one or more of the following:

- general state of physical health
- ability to reduce stress and anxiety
- nutrition state
- history of illness, past and present

Medical science has known since 1884 that alcohol abuse (excessive drinking, either in terms of amount or frequency, or in the effects of drinking on a given individual) results in reduced immunity to disease (MacGregor, p. 50). That is, drinking can reduce a person's ability to fight infectious diseases, including bacterial pneumonia, tuberculosis, and other viral or parasitic infections (MacGregor, p. 51). Laboratory research into the mechanisms and processes of the human immune system has shown that chemical abuse can have the following effects (individually or in combination):

- lowered resistance to disease
- reduced production of antibodies (which help fight disease)
- slowdown in the response rate in which the immune system reacts
- lowered ability to fight disease successfully (MacGregor, p. 53 *ff.*)

▪ ALCOHOL AND DRUG USE ▪ AND AIDS

Long before the effects of drug and alcohol use on the immune system can be observed, the influence of chemicals on behavior is obvious. In fact, it is often by observing another person's behavior that a caregiver may first become concerned and suspect drug and alcohol abuse.

Recent studies of persons with diagnoses of HIV infection, ARC, and AIDS reveal high percentages of drug and alcohol use (Seigel, p. 272). This is true among all populations: Caucasians, African Americans, Hispanics, et cetera. It is not limited to some other Them.

It has long been estimated that one out of every ten Americans is chemically dependent, that is to say, is physically and/or psychologically dependent on alcohol or other drugs. However, it is estimated that in the gay population, where AIDS first appeared in this country, three out of every ten persons have difficulties with alcohol or drugs (Seigel, p. 272).

Understand that alcohol and drug use does not *cause* infection with HIV. Mood-altering drugs may, however, be a cofactor. For the purposes of this discussion, a cofactor is anything that may play a role in determining who acquires HIV and whether or not the infection will progress to AIDS (Seigel, p. 272).

The biggest concerns that relate alcohol and drug use to HIV infection and the development of AIDS are these:

1. People who are drinking or drugging are more likely to engage in risky behavior (sexual or drug-related) that leads to HIV infection.
2. Persons with lowered immunity due to their previous alcohol and drug use may be more likely to become infected with HIV when first exposed.
3. Persons already infected with HIV may continue to destroy their immune system through drug and alcohol use.
4. Persons using alcohol or drugs may be more likely to participate in unsafe sexual behavior, increasing the risk that they will be exposed to HIV—or, if they are already exposed, that they will increase the risk of *transmitting* HIV to others or of becoming *reinfected* themselves.

▪ DEFINITION OF ▪
MOOD-ALTERING CHEMICALS

The use of mood-altering chemicals (so labeled because they have the capacity to chemically "change" human feelings) does not cause AIDS.

Rather, the use of:

- alcohol (beer, wine, liquor)
- marijuana
- stimulants (amphetamines, crystal, speed, cocaine, nicotine, caffeine)
- depressants (barbiturates, tranquilizers)
- opiates (heroin, morphine, codeine, methadone)

and any modifications of these substances are considered cofactors in the transmission and progression of HIV disease.

■ DEFINING DRUG USE AND ■ ALCOHOL ABUSE

As a caregiver, if you are uncertain about an individual's chemical use, but you suspect that the effects of alcohol or drugs may be influencing health or behavior, be assured that you are not alone. Even with experience and knowledge, it is often confusing and frustrating to try to determine what is really happening. More people with backgrounds in the field of substance-abuse counseling are providing care to those with HIV infection and offering support to their friends, partners, and family members.

The effects of drugs and alcohol may sometimes be mistaken for depression, the effects of other medications, or even AIDS-related dementia. Likewise, the effects of depression, medications, and dementia may sometimes be incorrectly ascribed to drug or alcohol use.

Whenever changes in behavior or pronounced changes in emotions or moods are observed, it is best for the caregiver to seek advice and clarification from a knowledgeable physician or counselor.

Some common behaviors that may indicate drug or alcohol use are:

- wide mood changes in short periods of time, several times a day; difficulty coping with intensity of feelings
- sudden changes from responsible to irresponsible behavior, poor motivation, lethargy, depression
- inability to follow through on commitments
- general faultfinding with all persons, especially with caregivers; externalizing all problems as the fault of others; seeking a "rescuer"
- the use of alcohol, drugs, or prescription medications, singly or in combination, to cope with any of the above

▪ DRUG AND ALCOHOL USE ▪ VERSUS ABUSE

It is important to note that an individual does not have to have a substance-abuse problem in order to use alcohol and drugs in ways that influence the ability of the immune system to fight disease.

In the same way, an individual does not have to abuse mood-altering chemicals in order for drugs and alcohol to affect behavior and relationships in negative ways.

Drug and alcohol *abuse* is defined as a pattern of "pathological use" that leads to a breakdown in an individual's relationships or ability to work, and that has a minimum duration of one month.

Pathological use is defined by at least one of the following:

- intoxication during the day (the effects of the drug or alcohol are felt and influence how a person acts)
- inability to decrease or stop drug or alcohol use (a person has tried to stop or to cut down but experiences a return to drugs or alcohol after a period of time)
- repeated attempts to control drug or alcohol use by cutting

down the amounts used, limiting how often the substance is used, and/or switching from one drug or one type of alcohol to another

- daily felt need for the drug or alcohol (either a felt emotional preoccupation or a physical urge)
- continued drug or alcohol use despite unpleasant consequences to health, relationships, or activity

Breakdown in relationships and job functioning is defined by:

- absence from work due to drug or alcohol use (flulike symptoms, hangovers, exhaustion, or "crashing"), or job performance influenced by effects of drug or alcohol use
- probation due to absence or poor work performance, loss of job, quitting job to avoid being fired, inability to hold a job for more than a few weeks or months, conflicts with co-workers or supervisors
- changes in mental abilities: loss of concentration, loss of memory (for shorter or longer periods of time), inability to think clearly or to make judgments, mood changes, inability to control impulses
- changes in behavior, such as increased irritability, aggression or depression, withdrawal from relationships, loss of motivation or self-esteem, compulsive behavior, increased irrational behavior
- problems with the law and/or increased conflicts with family or friends as a result of alcohol or drug use or the effects of alcohol or drug use (Levy)

It is not always easy to identify drug or alcohol abuse and its effects on health and behavior. If you are a caregiver and think you recognize some of the preceding characteristics in the behavior of someone you are caring for . . . or even in yourself . . . ask for the help and advice of someone who is experienced in the area of substance abuse or in the areas of drug and alcohol use and AIDS.

As a caregiver, there are some important facts to remember about the use of alcohol or drugs:

- Some people use alcohol and drugs with few adverse or negative effects to themselves or others.
- Pathological use of mood-altering chemicals is not your fault.
- Just as you did not cause the person you are caring for to drink or use drugs, neither can you control that person's use of mood-altering chemicals, nor make him/her stop.
- Drug and alcohol abuse can be motivated by a number of factors beyond a person's HIV infection or illness.
- Most abusers, in order to safely and successfully stop their drug and alcohol use and to stay abstinent, need the help and support of both professionals and people in recovery from substance abuse.

As a caregiver, you do not have to face the problem of drug abuse alone: There is help available to you and to the individual you are caring for.

In talking to someone with knowledge about substance abuse, describe what you have observed and what the person you are caring for may be experiencing. In some cases, the person you are caring for may be unaware of the effects of drugs or alcohol on his/her health and behavior. On the other hand, that individual may be frightened, unable, or unwilling to stop the use of mood-altering chemicals, with or without the help of professionals.

A knowledgeable doctor or counselor can help you become better informed about drug and alcohol use. He or she can also assist you in getting the help and support you need in order to make decisions about how you will communicate with and provide help to the person you are caring for.

▪ HOW TO TAKE CARE OF ▪ YOURSELF WHEN SOMEONE YOU ARE CARING FOR IS ABUSING DRUGS OR ALCOHOL

In order to better care for *yourself,* the following guidelines may give direction:

1. **SET YOUR LIMITS**

    If you do not wish to be around someone who is using drugs or alcohol, or who is high or seeking to use, say so—and then keep your word.

    Assure the person that you want to talk to and spend time with him/her, but only when the drug or alcohol use and its effects have stopped.

    If you decide not to be around someone who is using, go talk with a friend who can offer you support and encouragement *not* to rescue the person who is using. Al-Anon groups are a wonderful way to accomplish this: Call your local Alcoholics Anonymous group for information on Al-Anon.

2. **OFFER TO ASSIST THE PERSON TO GET MEDICAL HELP**

    If the person is seeking to obtain alcohol or drugs, or is physically uncomfortable because he/she is unable to find drugs or alcohol to use, or if you are being asked to supply mood-altering chemicals, offer instead to help the person get medical help.

    Never supply the person with drugs or alcohol or suggest the substitution of a prescription medication. Since you may not know what the person has used previously, additional drug use or the substitution of medications or alcohol can be dangerous.

In addition, if a person is in actual physical withdrawal from drug or alcohol use, he/she will need to be supervised by a physician.

3. BE SUPPORTIVE

A person suffering from drug or alcohol abuse will need your support, rather than your judgment, to cope with life. If the drug or alcohol use has become habitual, this person may need professional help to stop using.

You can be supportive without helping this person to continue using mood-altering chemicals. You can also learn to help without making excuses for or accepting behavior from this person that may be harmful to you.

4. BE HONEST

When discussing this person's drug or alcohol use with him/her, be honest and specific. "You always . . ." is not specific; "Last Monday afternoon you . . ." is.

Refer to specific times of drug/alcohol use and the ways in which this person's behavior affected you. Describe how you *feel,* rather than what you may *think,* about this person's behavior.

Encourage the person to talk about his/her feelings also.

5. BE AWARE OF YOUR OWN DRUG OR ALCOHOL USAGE

Caregivers are also prone to drug and alcohol misuse. Watch yourself and seek counseling if you feel (or are told) that you are slipping.

6. *REMEMBER THAT YOU ARE NOT ALONE*

If you need help to deal with an alcohol or drug-abusing person, or if the person expresses a desire to get help, remember that there are a number of community resources that can assist both of you.

The locations and numbers of the following resources can usually be found in the telephone book or by calling Directory Assistance. In smaller communities, you may be able to locate services in the nearest larger city or through area or county agencies.

▪ Alcoholics Anonymous and Narcotics Anonymous: These peer-support-group meetings are held on a regular basis. Meetings are cost-free and are designed to help people stay abstinent from drugs and alcohol by using a Twelve Step program. Some AA and NA groups also provide support to HIV-infected persons through specific meetings that address recovery and HIV infection.

▪ Al-Anon, Nar-Anon, Codependents Anonymous, Adult Children of Alcoholics: These peer-support-group meetings are also held regularly for the spouses, partners, friends, and children of alcoholics and drug addicts. They focus on self-care, detachment, and self-esteem.

▪ A local city or county Council on Alcoholism and Drug Abuse: Such agencies provide information on drug and alcohol abuse, counseling and treatment programs, free evaluation services, and regular education programs.

▪ Local or area AIDS service agencies may be able to provide you with additional information on drug and alcohol use and AIDS, as well as programs for education, counseling, and support for persons seeking help, both those with HIV illnesses and their caregivers.

• GETTING AND STAYING •
SOBER

A common misconception is that persons who are HIV infected do not want to stop drinking or using drugs.

I have heard people say, "If I had AIDS, I'd want to keep on using. Why get sober if you're going to die anyway?"

The truth is, there *are* men and women who choose to cope with HIV infection by drinking and taking drugs. But there are also many men and women with HIV infection who have chosen to get sober—and are staying abstinent—in order to live more fully and healthier than ever before.

There are good reasons for their choice:

- Sobriety can give the immune system a chance to work on its own, without the added stress of alcohol and drug use.
- Alcohol and drug use can sometimes interfere in the benefits of medicines; abstinence permits the body to receive the full benefit of any medical preventative or treatment therapy for HIV illness.
- Abstinence gives individuals the opportunity to make clearer, better-informed decisions about what they truly want from life, unobstructed by the legal, financial, family, and job problems caused by chemical use.

The decision to stop drug and alcohol use is not an easy one. Staying sober from alcohol or straight from drugs is not easily achieved. That is why support from caregivers and others in chemical recovery is so important to the HIV-infected individual.

As an AIDS caregiver, you have the right to be informed about the relationship between drug and alcohol use and AIDS as it affects those you care about.

It is important for you to know that you are not alone, that information and help are available to you if you are at all concerned about the drug or alcohol use of someone you take care of or provide assistance to.

In addition to knowing the characteristics of substance abuse, it is crucial for you to find sound advice for yourself when dealing with a substance-abusing person. In addition to understanding how drug and alcohol use can influence health and behavior, it is also vital for you to know how to support the person you are caring for while setting reasonable limits, so that the helping relationship you share can be a healthy one.

▪ BIBLIOGRAPHY ▪

Levy, Ronald. *The New Language of Psychiatry: Learning and Using DSM-III.* Boston: Little, Brown, and Company, 1982.

MacGregor, Rob Roy. "Alcohol and Drugs as Co-factors for AIDS," *AIDS and Substance Abuse,* ed. Larry Seigel. New York: The Hawthorne Press, 1988.

Scott, Neil. "AIDS, Alcohol, and Drugs," *Alcoholism and Addiction,* May-June 1988, pp. 14–16.

Seigel, Larry. "AIDS: Relationships to Alcohol and Other Drugs," *The Journal of Substance Abuse Treatment,* Vol. 3 (1986), pp. 271–74.

19

▪STORIES FROM▪ THE FRONT: PROVIDING A HOME TO A DRUG ABUSER

AN INTERVIEW WITH DON MAISON

Dallas attorney Don Maison is Executive Director of AIDS Services of Dallas. Previous to becoming the agency's first Executive Director in February 1989, Don was a trial lawyer in a private firm and was actively involved in litigating issues affecting the rights of HIV-infected individuals. He remains active in that forum, as his time permits.

EIDSON: Will you give us an overview of the types of services your agency provides to people living with AIDS?

MAISON: We provide medically supportive housing for low-income and indigent individuals and families living with symptomatic AIDS/HIV disease. We began in 1987 and have housed more than three hundred individuals and families, providing more than fifty-five thousand person-nights of care. We currently house more than sixty individuals in two large facilities. We offer twenty-four-hour on-site home care, substance-abuse-recovery support service, food and household furnishings as available, and we work with other resources to fill in any gaps in service.

EIDSON: Among the persons who have received services, have you encountered drug abusers in the populations seeking housing?

MAISON: Absolutely. Active drug users in congregate housing can destroy a program, and maintaining a drug-free environment requires a great deal of vigilance, professional intervention, and support.

EIDSON: In terms of drug users, what has been the worst experience you have had?

MAISON: The worst? First, in clarifying what you mean by that, I have learned a great deal out here in the trenches I would not otherwise have known. When you use the term "drug user" in reference to the population we serve, I tend to immediately think of injectible drug users (IDUs) because of my experiences with those persons who engage in that behavior. I was pretty ignorant about those behaviors when I first took over here.

My perception is colored by the types of things that happened to other residents because of that type of addictive behavior. There were some pretty egregious things that occurred and that we learned about only after the fact. Fortunately, we have a licensed social worker on our staff now who helps with our screening process and our recovering populations, and that has provided us the skill to intervene promptly when problems do occur.

But the worst experience, as you put it, is probably our Star of Stage and Screen: a resident who has been featured in the newspapers; who was touted in the press as "Mr. Person Living with AIDS." He had been flown all around the country to talk with young people about HIV disease and was generally perceived to be quite the spokesperson on HIV-related issues. I recall that at a staff meeting, I learned that six rigs had been found in his bathroom, lined up from a party the night before. That was a shocking occurrence to me, partly because I was let down by my own perceptions of this individual. I was pretty street-stupid then. In fact, that was when I first learned what the term "rig" meant.

But as I think about my experiences over the past three years, I don't know that I could characterize that as the most egregious. I would say the most horrible experiences are where the behaviors result in the victimization of people who are less able to care for themselves. There is one such occasion that comes to mind:

We had an active IDU in our program who had stolen our property—specifically, microwave ovens—and sold them in the neighborhood to crack dealers; he pawned other residents' property and our property; and he stole medications from other clients. And we caught him dealing! We learned all of these behaviors during the course of a couple of hours. This was long before we had social workers on staff. After we found out about the microwaves, all this other stuff began coming out about this person; but something had to occur to break the code of silence, so to speak.

Our residents' council was still developing then; there wasn't a great sense of being empowered to control one's existence or environment. I would also characterize the situation as one of helplessness for the residents, in terms of whom staff would agree to bring into the program and impose on their lives.

What's different now is that in addition to having professional staff on-site to assist with screening and support, our residents' council now participates in the actual screening process for prospective residents. They go through a series of questions that staff has negotiated with them: I wanted them asking relevant questions that were pertinent to congregate-living issues, not about race or religion, et cetera. We now have some clear-cut standards by which residents have an important role in deciding who is going to be in the same housing program with them. It's appropriate. And so far it has been dynamic. There has been what I perceive to be a sense of responsibility for what goes on in terms of appropriate behaviors, which has been healthy for residents and staff alike.

We didn't always have that structure. It was just developing in the fall of 1989. Supportive housing did not receive adequate funding in those days (and it still doesn't, for that matter), and we had only five people on staff for a client population that hovered around thirty at that time.

EIDSON: Tell me what happened. What brought the thefts and dealing situations to your attention?

MAISON: I was fortunate to have gotten a former resident on staff. We hired Victor to be Facilities Manager, and his credentials were superb.

Victor had had his own experiences with drugs, and he overcame them. When he sought a staff position, I wanted him to move off-property, for his own sanity. He was popular as a resident and was an important part of the push to involve residents in decision making concerning prospective residents.

Victor came to our agency in the spring of 1989. Our residents' manager, Judith, came to me rather upset. She said, "Well, it finally happened." I said, "What happened?" She informed me that we had had our first referral from the Texas Board of Pardons and Paroles. I remember sitting here, incredibly busy at that moment, and I asked why she was upset. "I don't know what to do!" she said.

I told her she had given me no information: "Are we talking

about a Charles Manson? Or are we talking about somebody who jaywalked too many times and didn't pay their fine?" (I wasn't sure at that time whether our then tiny and overworked staff even understood the distinction between the Probation Department and the Board of Pardons and Paroles.) There was a clear sense of relief on her part: She sensed permission to investigate further.

Keep in mind that our process of admission had not developed into what it is today, and that we were trying to be very careful about whom we were putting into congregate living situations, because we had encountered some big problems that were gradually being remedied. During 1989 we were extremely understaffed, overworked, and underfunded.

One morning I came in late. (I had a docket I had to meet, and during the first months of my job, I had to complete some legal obligations I had to clients. So there were some mornings I would have to be in court before going to the agency.) I walked into the front door of our then primitive office and observed this man on a ladder texturing walls. I did a double take and thought, "I don't remember authorizing anyone to hire a contractor to fix our offices." I was perplexed.

Mike Anderson, the Program Director (who is now our Assistant Executive Director), was nearby. I said, "What the hell's going on here? Who is paying this guy?"

Anderson said, "No, no, you don't understand. This is Judith's idea of a test."

"I beg your pardon?"

He said, "Remember that guy she asked you about?"

I'm sure I remarked that I had slept several times since then and that I didn't remember.

He reminded me about the referral from the Texas Board of Pardons and Paroles, and my memory was jogged.

"Well, she looked into it and talked with him, and she liked him, but she wasn't sure he wasn't conning, so she gave him a 'test.' "

I remarked that I thought it was absurd to give people "tests" like this for admission. It was only later I would come to respect some very fundamental assessment skills of someone who had been in this business longer than I and had worked more closely with the populations we were beginning to serve.

Well, to make a long story short, he finished his task. He won Judith's heart; she believed that he would be most appropriate as a resident; and he moved in. He was my first experience with a resident who understood what empowerment was all about. He looked at his room and said he thought it was dingy. (It was: The place was ugly.) "It needs a paint job; it needs to be textured." And he bought his materials, got his own roller, textured his walls, and fixed up his room. Then he showed Jeff how to do it; Jeff showed Tom how to do it; Tom showed Joey how to do it. . . . All of a sudden we had seven rooms in that facility that were freshly textured and painted. So needless to say, he was quite an impressive resident.

And his story is probably not atypical for a lot of HIV-infected people, that is, *after* they go through an initial stage of denial and anger.

In Victor's case, he learned he was HIV infected in California; then he was diagnosed with ARC. He went through what I conclude is a typical experience: "I have HIV. Deny and be angry." Victor returned to Dallas. Victor partied big time. He got busted in his family's home. He got a year to do because he resisted arrest. He's off parole now. Coming to us gave him a chance to make a new life for himself.

Victor managed the renovation of our second facility, a twenty-eight-unit complex adjacent to our first, and now he manages both our properties as part of staff. His perspective as a former resident is very important.

But, back to our crime problem. Victor is more streetwise than I am. He can sniff out drug-related behavior like nobody I have ever known. He had been spending a great deal of time at our second facility, getting ready for the rehabilitation project we had just been funded for; he noticed a stranger leaving this guy's unit carrying a microwave, going from our facility into the tenement next door.

Victor followed this guy into a neighboring complex in which one of our neighborhood plumbers lived. (Hiring locals was one way we made and kept friends in the neighborhood, you see.) So Victor talked to our plumber, Tony. Tony became our spy and found out from his neighbor that the microwave had been exchanged for drugs.

Mike, Victor, and I all went to confront our resident with the information we had learned. James, our resident, said that he had sent the microwave off for repairs. Then Victor looked at James's stereo: It was another resident's, Calvin's. It turned out that James had stolen Calvin's stereo.

That was a real fact-finding mission. Shortly thereafter, our entire staff of six went to visit. By that time, James had passed out on his couch, surrounded by empty medication bottles from other, more medically compromised, clients. He was strung out: I only thought he was having a bad day! Victor wised me up. I gave James two hours to get out.

A year later, we received a letter from him, written a day or two before he died—an incredible letter wanting to make peace, and apologizing for falling back into crack-cocaine use. But he went on to say that he understood that we had to do what we had to do, and that he concurred with our decision because he had been a threat to other residents. He had been out of control, and admitted it in his letter. It was so sad. He wrote to assure us that we had done more for him than we would ever realize. It was a mind-blowing letter.

EIDSON: I'm listening to you from the perspective of a parent who comes in and finds his son or daughter has stolen from him. It's a common occurrence with parents housing kids who are drug users. What do you do then? The answer is: You throw the creep out—NOW! Regardless if it is your son or daughter. Then how do you deal with the guilt? Your letter from the now deceased drug dealer is the answer: Here is a guy who has come back from his deathbed and said, "What you did was right, and thank you."

MAISON: He did that. We have a file of letters from residents who are now deceased, parents of residents who have died, friends and lovers of former residents who, in their own way, each say the same thing. Mostly letters saying, "Thank you for being tough with me, and for keeping the place a safe place to live."

EIDSON: That was your worst scenario, even though it has a happy ending. Now, what do you feel has been your best scenario with a drug user?

MAISON: Well, we have no best scenario with an active drug user. Only problems. (We're not, of course, talking about medication drugs, but illicit drugs.) We haven't had any good experiences with active drug users. We have had very positive experiences with people who were addicts and who desired a supportive environment to facilitate recovery.

EIDSON: Let's look at that. If someone were going to be starting some kind of a housing facility and they knew that they were going to be getting drug users, what would you tell them?

MAISON: I'd tell them not to. Don't get me wrong; we house heroin addicts. But we provide them with an environment that is supportive toward *recovery from addiction.* You can't provide housing to an integrated population without systems in place to support recovery, in my opinion. I've seen too much not to believe that addictions lead to victimizing weaker persons toward whom we have a special obligation.

There are a number of times we have discovered *active* drug use in our applicant-screening process. And also in reviewing our prospective clients' histories. The best advice I could give someone contemplating something like that is: Yes, we respect individual freedom; yes, we believe that people should be able to do what they want, et cetera; but the fact of the matter is that you are dealing with a sick population needing essential services, and there isn't enough money to provide a staff-to-client ratio to protect the vulnerable. So we continue to deal with dual diagnoses: HIV and substance abuse. That reality will impede a program if it isn't dealt with frankly.

Simply stated, what we do is open our doors to anyone who is *recovering* from injectible drug use or other drug or alcohol abuse, or to those who agree to set goals or get into a program, as facts warrant on an individual basis. We require those with injectible-drug-abuse histories to demonstrate that they are in an acceptable drug-rehabilitation program. As part of our agreement with each resident, we ask that they will agree to a drug test at any time at our request. If they decline the test, they're out. If they test positive, they either agree to get into individual or group programs approved by our social worker, or they're out. If they are negative on a test, we pay for it. We have utilized our drug-testing policy perhaps four times in the past year. Just having the policy in place has been an important tool to supportive recovery, in my opinion.

Our happiest-ending story is probably a married couple with a history of IDU who got into a methadone program: Her health improved; they had a child. He went through vocational rehab and was employed as a photocopier technician. She was employed by another AIDS-service organization in town. They saved their money, got their own house, and have been doing well for the past few years. I would consider that a story with a happy ending.

There are other stories with happy endings as well. And I certainly don't mean to imply that it's impossible to provide housing to a population with a history of drug abuse; but I can state that there is no way you can mix an *active* drug-using population with an HIV housing program. You have to be willing to deal with an IDU very directly, very firmly, and very supportively. The problem is always watching out for those who are medically compromised, because active IDUs tend to stop at nothing to support their addiction. These situations were new to my experience when I started.

EIDSON: That's a good response to people who might be thinking of starting a program. But what would you tell parents who are thinking of taking in a family member who has a history of drug use?

MAISON: I believe the message is the same for a family member or loved one: If they are *active* IDUs, the answer is NO! The advice I would give to parents, brothers, sisters, or loved ones who might be prone to rescue—and I think most of us are —is to be firm on insisting that the IDU get help from professionals in a recovery program. I believe this is an important step that must be taken before agreeing to house the individual. I know that is easier said than done. I have a friend whose son has taken him for thousands, drained bank accounts, charged credit cards to the max, and pawned household items to support a cocaine habit. My friend rescued his son so many times that it was frustrating for me to stand by and watch them both self-destruct.

As a practical matter, I recall one person who applied for housing here and we could not accommodate him. He was diagnosed with AIDS, and he was an active IDU. He declined to get into recovery. We referred him to the Salvation Army for shelter, where he lived for about eight months, until his health had declined to the point we refer to as Level Four, or terminal phase. He was too close to death at that point to be out on the streets, and we let him in toward the final weeks of his life. That's a rather grim but possible scenario for active IDUs who can be accommodated, but only when they are too ill or too close to death to be able to be much of a threat to others.

To a parent I would say that if an AIDS-diagnosed child will not get into active recovery (and that recovery would more than likely require participation by the parent or parents and all the commitments that requires), the other option would be to intervene at the terminal phase of the disease. That sounds pretty grim, but it is likely the only feasible point at which intervention would be possible. I say this, of course, from the experiences I have had in real-life situations, particularly in working with IDUs who are part of the population of persons living with AIDS that we serve, and not as a professional drug-abuse expert.

It has taken us a while to acquire the skills to be able to deal effectively and fairly with populations this disease has affected epidemiologically, who have been thrown together by its impact. We are encountering a larger number of IDUs in AIDS care and services, and it's not exactly the same kind of single-front battle. We have had to learn how to access other service providers . . . and there are pitifully few around here that will provide help to this population. We have a few; they, too, are underfunded and are having to learn about AIDS as AIDS caregivers are learning about IDUs.

But caregivers are having to learn about people, and that is really what is happening in this epidemic. Just look at our client population: In February 1989, when I started here, it was an entirely Caucasian, entirely gay, male population. And although Dallas continues to lead the nation in AIDS-diagnosed cases in the Caucasian gay male community, our client census has had a mixture of at least 25 percent women and children, and 35 percent racial and ethnic minorities for the past couple of years.

We've had to develop some new skills in working with all these different populations in a congregate housing community of people living with AIDS. But in so many ways, it is just like the real world is. And it takes some experience to overcome the myths we all harbored about IDUs and to learn to like and respect them for who they are. After all, someone who has been an IDU and wants to come into our program is showing us the courage and commitment to deal with a dual diagnosis: That's tough, and that person has my respect and my support in all the ways we've talked about.

20

·WOMEN·
AND HIV DISEASE

BARBARA S. CAMBRIDGE, PH.D., A.C.S.W., C.S.W.-A.C.P.
(in collaboration with Madeline, Susie, Kim, E.J., and Norma)

Dr. Cambridge is an Associate Professor in the Department of Obstetrics and Gynecology at Southwestern Medical Center in Dallas, Texas. She is the coordinator of the Women's Support Services for the Pediatric HIV Health Care Demonstration Project (HRSA) and the founder and leader of the Women Educating Women Team, a group of HIV-infected women who work with other infected women, touring statewide and sharing their stories and experiences. She has been facilitating support groups for women with HIV disease since 1987.

If you are reading this chapter, I suspect you are involved or contemplating involvement in the care of women living with HIV disease. Good: This chapter is written especially for you. In choosing to provide care and support for women, all kinds of feelings surface. Men sometimes feel anxious and uncomfortable about working with women, especially sick women. Individuals of different racial and economic backgrounds may also feel unsure about the most effective way to be of support. Relax; I'm here to tell you that all of your feelings, emotions, and concerns are normal and appropriate. After reading this chapter, you will have gained, I hope, some understanding about the role you can play in "walking the path" with women living with HIV disease.

· HISTORICAL PERSPECTIVE ·

Women have been a part of the AIDS epidemic since the beginning, although failure to diagnose and adequately report cases among them may be a major factor in their low statistical representation. At the very least, women represent 12 percent of all diagnosed cases. (Although African Americans and Latinos make up only 19 percent of the general population, they provide 70 percent of the reported cases among women.) Women represent one of the fastest-growing populations affected by HIV disease, which is now the fifth-leading cause of death among women between the ages of fifteen and forty-four. Some estimates suggest that more that eighty thousand women in the United States are already infected with HIV but undiagnosed.

· WHO ARE THESE WOMEN? ·

- Myra, thirty-one years old, attractive, the manager of a fashionable ladies' boutique, was diagnosed after her twelve-year marriage to a bisexual man ended.
- Today Kitty celebrates her fifteenth birthday. Kitty has been a prostitute for two years and has full-blown AIDS.
- Senora, sixty-one, enjoys her grandchildren's weekend visits, but she is terrified their parents will learn of her infection and restrict her involvement with the children.

▪ Angela and Mark have been married five years and have two children, three-year-old Mike and eighteen-month-old Sissy. The marriage has always been troubled because of Mark's drug use. Repeated conflicts with Angela's family have resulted in alienation. Angela, Mark, Mike, and little Sissy have all been diagnosed with HIV disease.

▪ Kate received several blood transfusions after the birth of her second child. No one knew the blood was contaminated.

Women affected by HIV disease represent a wide range of ethnic, racial, social, educational, and economic backgrounds. They are mothers, daughters, wives, lovers, grandmothers, sisters, aunts. They are religious and nonreligious. They are inner-city drug users, prostitutes, high school and college students, and suburban housewives. Of particular concern is the growing number of adolescent girls, aged twelve to seventeen, who are being diagnosed. These young women, with their unique social, psychological, and developmental issues, may represent a population for whom a new model of care will be necessary.

▪ HOW WERE THEY INFECTED? ▪

This is a question frequently asked by persons becoming involved with HIV-infected women. A majority of these women contracted the virus through one of three primary means: intravenous drug use (50 percent); sexual contact with an infected partner (27 percent); or contaminated blood (less than 10 percent).

Female partners of bisexual men, IV-drug users, and hemophiliacs are at particularly high risk of becoming infected. While more men than women carry the virus, women vastly outnumber men in infection through heterosexual contact. (Although the presence of the virus has been found to exist in the vaginal secretion of infected women, the risk of female-to-male transmission is significantly lower than that of male-to-female transmission.) It is not uncommon for women to be unaware of changes within the vagina (minor cuts, abrasions, open lesions). Such conditions may allow the virus to enter the woman's bloodstream during unprotected vaginal sex. The same is true for unprotected oral and anal sexual activities.

New blood-screening techniques have significantly reduced the risk of receiving contaminated blood or blood products. Early in the epidemic, at least 10 percent of women contracted the virus through contaminated transfusions.

The means of infection is a sensitive issue for many women. Some perceive any question on the subject as the basis for stereotyping and making moral judgments. Unless your need to know will affect your participation in an HIV-infected woman's care, respect her privacy and wait until she chooses to share the information.

Shirley, a woman in our support group, puts it this way: "It really doesn't matter how you got it; how you live with it is what counts."

• CLINICAL MANIFESTATION •

Females, especially women of childbearing age, have traditionally been excluded from large clinical studies and drug trials. Because of this, it is only from anecdotal and informal data that we believe that HIV disease in women is significantly different than in men. There is only limited formal data regarding HIV-disease progression in women and the virus's impact on a woman's general health. Though some knowledge exists about the affect of the women's hormones on her overall immune system, there is almost no information about the added affect of HIV.

Having said this, it might be helpful to identify some signs and symptoms associated with HIV infection in women. Please be aware, however, that these symptoms may also appear in uninfected women.

- recurring yeast infections
- abdominal pain unrelated to menstrual period
- unusual vaginal discharge
- open sores, lesions on the genitals
- repeated and unresponsive sexually transmitted disease (STD) history
- abnormal Pap results
- swollen glands (neck, armpit, groin) that last for several weeks or longer
- severe weight loss without dieting
- night sweats
- white, patchy coating on tongue or elsewhere in the mouth (thrush)
- chronic fatigue
- prolonged periods of diarrhea

▪ CONCERNS AND ISSUES ▪

The diagnosis of HIV disease affects not only the woman with the illness but also her entire family. Women with HIV disease are usually living within some family unit (related or unrelated by blood). Some are single, some are single mothers, and some are married or living in a relationship with a significant other.

Let's explore some issues and concerns HIV-infected women face.

▪ HEALTH CARE AND PERSONAL ▪ WELLNESS

For many women, obtaining competent, confidential health care is very difficult. It is not uncommon for a woman to seek medical care for recurring health problems over a period of several years before finally receiving an HIV diagnosis. (The diagnosis is usually made after the woman changes health-care providers, becomes pregnant, or experiences a medical crisis.) Once diagnosed, some women and their family members are required to seek care elsewhere. This is particularly true for women in small rural communities where accessible health care is limited or nonexistent. Limited access forces many women to seek care in larger nearby cities or to go without care until a crisis develops.

Recently, we attempted to help a woman locate a gynecologist who would care for an HIV-positive woman on Medicaid. After numerous calls, we located a physician who would accept Medicaid payments but would not accept HIV patients, and a physician who would treat HIV patients but would not accept Medicaid payments. This is not a problem men generally have to face.

Caregivers can help by encouraging women to obtain early preventative health care and to adopt healthy life-styles. Other support activities include:

- teaching a woman to ask questions and keep track of information obtained during clinic visits
- encouraging her to ask questions
- serving as her advocate during medical visits
- sharing information clipped from timely and reliable publications

Once enrolled in a good, supportive health-care system, HIV-infected women seem to do as well as HIV-infected men. Again, the key here is connecting with a competent, female-friendly care system committed to serving women living with HIV disease.

▪ FEAR ▪

HIV-infected women often feel particularly vulnerable. They fear for their own well-being and that of their children. They may fear the loss of family support more strongly than men. Mothers may be concerned about the safety and acceptance of their children both at school and within the family. For these reasons immediate family members are sometimes the last to know of the diagnosis and often are informed only when a medical crisis demands disclosure.

A care provider must be sensitive to these issues and maintain confidentiality. Never assume that family members or significant others are aware of the diagnosis. Any conversations regarding the nature of a woman's health should be strictly between you and your primary client.

▪ SEXUAL INTIMACY ▪

For many women, the childhood dream of a happy marriage, children, a nice home, and a career is just that: a dream. HIV disease forces a woman to reevaluate and possibly to make dramatic changes in her social/sexual behavior. HIV-infected women often raise these questions: What am I going to do about sex? Am I to remain celibate for the remainder of my life? Will anyone want to date or become involved with a person like me? Though I am healthy now, do I have a right to enter a relationship, knowing that I might become sick, create a financial burden on my partner, and, ultimately, die?

A woman's own response to these questions will depend largely on her present coping skills, her capacity to acquire additional skills, and the degree of support she receives from others. Some women will choose to reexamine their life-style, sexuality, and value system, and seek new ways of living. Other women will respond by denying the reality of their infection and will continue life as usual. Unfortunately, a number of women, because of fear of rejection, choose to respond to HIV infection by withdrawing socially, creating a form of social imprisonment. Women with a history of depression or drug use may escape into such unhelpful coping patterns.

Gloria, a woman living with HIV disease, says that for her, "Having AIDS feels like having a giant *A* stamped on my forehead, making me unlovable, undesirable, and unavailable."

Making regular personal contact (visits or telephone calls), encouraging the use of confidential AIDS hot lines, sharing information about available services (support groups, professional counseling), and offering to accompany a woman to a support-group meeting are just a few things that caregivers may do to help decrease the sense of isolation and loneliness experienced by HIV-infected women.

■ REPRODUCTIVE DECISIONS ■

The question of childbearing is one of the most complex dilemmas any woman faces, but it is especially complicated for HIV-infected women (the majority of whom are of childbearing age). The potential acceleration of the disease during pregnancy and the possibility of perinatal transmission are serious considerations. Other considerations include: Will I inflict pain and suffering on my child? Could this be my only/last chance to have a child with my partner? Who will provide care for me and my child if we both are ill? Will I die before my child reaches maturity? Do I have a right to impose this situation on my other children, my family?

Early in the AIDS epidemic, women were counseled of a 100 percent risk of mother-to-child transmission. Based on this advice, many women chose pregnancy termination. Currently, women are advised that perinatal transmission is only about a 20 to 30 percent likelihood. Some women consider this a relatively small risk, while others feel that 20 percent is still too big a chance to take.

Many women's diagnosis of HIV infection is made during pregnancy, and they must wait several months after delivery before a definitive diagnosis can be made for the baby. (A newborn child is born with the mother's antibodies to HIV, regardless if the child itself is HIV infected. See Chapter 17 on pediatrics.)

An HIV-infected mother *is* capable of giving birth to an uninfected infant. Unfortunately, at this time, health-care professionals are unable to determine which pregnancies will be affected. As research efforts are increased, this kind of information will become available.

For a variety of reasons, women *do* choose to bear children in spite of the uncertainty. Reproductive decisions for HIV-infected women are, at the very least, complex and highly emotional. As a caregiver, your ability to be a good listener, a sounding board, and a confidant will be extremely valuable. Respect for a woman's decision is of primary importance. It is inappropriate and unsupportive to attempt to impose your own personal values and beliefs in this situation.

▪ FINANCIAL STABILITY ▪

The financial security of her family is another major area of concern for an HIV-infected woman. Regardless of her marital status, an infected woman's need to provide for her family is a tremendous burden on her.

Excessive absenteeism due to personal or family illness may jeopardize a woman's employment. Employer's sick-leave policies may require written verification of the nature of the illness, and failure to satisfy this requirement may be cause for termination. Again, the issue of disclosure is raised.

Although repeated gynecological problems may render a woman unable to maintain regular employment, she is often denied access to government disability programs because gynecological problems are not considered by the Centers for Disease Control to be opportunistic infections. As more clinical studies are opened to women and sufficient data are gathered about disease manifestation in women, this issue will be resolved.

▪ INSURANCE COVERAGE ▪

Historically, the population affected by HIV disease (mostly young people) is unaccustomed to obtaining adequate insurance coverage. Most insurance coverage is employment-connected. For the unemployed or under-employed, private coverage is either too expensive or simply unavailable. Future financial security becomes a real dilemma for mothers with dependent children.

Marsha, age twenty-nine, recently diagnosed with AIDS, mother of three young children, was fired from her job because of excessive absenteeism due to her illness. Her job loss resulted in termination of her insurance coverage. Marsha expresses concern about dying and leaving her children the expenses associated with her funeral. But her most pressing worry is the financial care of her children after her death.

■ WOMEN AS CAREGIVERS ■

Women are generally socialized to assume responsibility for the care of family members. Providing care for a sick child, significant other, or other family members may be doubly difficult for an HIV-infected person. Then, if the sick family members are themselves HIV-infected, the task becomes almost insurmountable. In addition to being a mother, wife, and lover with HIV disease, she must also assume the roles of nurse, pharmacist, physician's assistant, interpreter, in-home case manager, family advocate, and negotiator. The family's physical and emotional wellness depends heavily on a woman's ability to perform all these jobs, but the Superwoman role can have a devastating effect on an HIV-infected woman's own health. All too often, the woman is so consumed with ensuring adequate care for her family that she neglects her own care.

■ OTHER WOMEN AFFECTED ■ BY HIV DISEASE

Uninfected women in relationships with infected persons are yet another group of persons living with HIV disease: They are wives, lovers, mothers, daughters, siblings, and caregivers. Many of the issues affecting HIV-infected woman are of concern to this group as well: for instance, decisions regarding children, financial security, and handling the expanded role of family provider.

Her infected partner may withdraw from sexual activity, even completely safe sex practices, due to the fear of infecting her. Too, large doses of daily medications, chronic fatigue, depression, and grieving may cause the infected partner to lose sexual desire. In either case the withdrawal of the partner sexually can create a tremendous emotional burden for the woman. Living with HIV disease requires a couple to openly communicate their concerns and fears, and to seek new ways of meeting their emotional and sexual needs. Couples experiencing intimacy problems are encouraged to seek counseling.

▪ WHO ARE A WOMAN'S ▪ CAREGIVERS?

▪ FAMILY OF ORIGIN ▪

Housing, financial assistance, and nursing care may be provided by parents, older children, and adult siblings. For many women, however, having to depend heavily on family members for support because of a shift in financial circumstances and/or declining health status is a tremendous blow to self-worth and independence. Such arrangements, although necessary, can place considerable strain on family relationships.

▪ HUSBANDS AND MALE PARTNERS ▪

Generally speaking, men feel less able than women to handle the duties of a caregiver within a family situation. The skills have not been traditionally taught to men in our society. Lack of knowledge may be exacerbated by feelings of guilt and helplessness if the man believes he may be responsible for bringing the virus into the family.

Many men, however, rise to the occasion and become the most valuable caregivers. This will depend not on the man's socioeconomic status as much as on his own life lessons. His childhood and young adult experiences of illness, death, and grief will influence his response to his own family's need.

Other caregivers need to be careful not to judge a male partner's level of commitment to the care of his infected female partner and children. Many men assume the role of primary caregiver and, with adequate support from both family and outsiders, perform the job admirably.

▪ SIGNIFICANT OTHERS ▪

Other people—lovers, roommates (both male and female), co-workers, and friends—should not be excluded from the list of potential caregivers. For many women, this array of significant others forms the basis for a surrogate family-support system.

▪ THE CHURCH AS CAREGIVER ▪

Religious institutions have, for whatever reasons, often missed opportunities to provide significant support to individuals and families in crisis in their communities, sometimes within their own congregations. Some women have reported being asked to leave congregations because of their HIV-positive status. The good news, however, is that more and more churches, synagogues, and meetinghouses are demonstrating a willingness to carry their ministries beyond their own walls, and now offer care services designed to decrease a woman's feelings of loneliness, depression, and social isolation. They affirm the value of the person and provide multiple support alternatives: they develop programs that seek to expand AIDS education beyond their own

292 • AIDS CAREGIVER'S HANDBOOK

congregations; they become involved in community coalitions established to create and expand needed health and social services for HIV-infected women and their families.

The list of specific service opportunities open to church-based groups is endless, and includes:

- participation in "mother's day out" and other existing child-care programs
- assistance with basic living needs (food, shelter, clothing)
- assistance with home health-care needs
- home baby-sitting
- pastoral care and counseling, especially in the area of funeral planning

One urban church's experience involved Nancy, a single woman with HIV disease in her mid-twenties. Nancy had accepted the imminence of her death and had made her own funeral arrangements; she gained permission to use the church for the service and asked the minister to conduct it. A member of the congregation encouraged and assisted her to attend Sunday services for as long as she was physically able to do so. While other church members were uncomfortable with Nancy's presence, a small core of men and women were able to reach out to her. Eventually, Nancy asked if she could be baptized. Her request was granted, and on the Sunday of her baptism she arrived at the church smiling brightly, wearing a lovely dress and corsage provided by one of her supporters. Amid a chorus of friends and fellow congregants, she received the sacrament of baptism; afterward, some of the churchwomen gave a reception in her honor.

The congregation continued its outreach, making weekly visits and telephone calls, preparing Nancy's favorite foods, feeding her, and offering daily prayers for her. Less than six weeks after Nancy's baptismal celebration, friends and church members returned to the church for her funeral service.

Yes, there were members of this congregation who remained uncomfortable, but they were in a small minority.

The impact that religious institutions can have on easing the burden of women and families living and dying with terminal diseases like AIDS is profound.

■ CONCLUSION ■

I hope that reading this chapter has significantly increased your level of comfort about becoming a caregiver for women. If you bring to the task your unique personality and life experience, your willingness and commitment to help, I am confident that your own life and the lives of the women you support will be greatly enriched.

·AFTERWORD:·
WHERE ARE
THEY NOW?

The Oak Lawn Counseling Center changed its name to Oak Lawn Community Services to better explain its diversity. Its new address is P.O. Box 191094, Dallas, Texas 75219.

Dr. Charles Haley, M.D., M.S., F.A.C.S., remains with the Dallas County Health Department.

Dr. Brady Allen, M.D., still practices medicine in Dallas.

Dr. Alan Hamill, D.O., also continues his practice in Dallas.

Jack Hamilton, C.S.W.-A.C.P., and **Vicki Morris, R.N., M.S.W., L.P.C.,** are now exclusively in private practice in the Dallas area. Both are active in seminar presentations, Jack specializing in wellness issues, and Vicki in women's empowerment.

Amelia London continues to live in Dallas, spending more time with her surviving children and their families, and less time with the parents' groups she helped establish, of which there are now several.

Candice J. Marcum, M.Ed., L.P.C., has a Dallas practice that has grown toward family and marriage issues.

Billy Burton, who was diagnosed with AIDS in 1983, continues to live in good health, with continuing immuno-deficiency-related ailments that no one has heard of before (the downside of being a long-term survivor). He has moved from Dallas to South Padre Island, Texas, where he can enjoy the beach year-round. He has resigned from most of his board activities to spend time with the things in life he most enjoys.

David H. Stout, A.C.S.W., C.S.W.-A.C.P., left Oak Lawn Counseling Center in November 1989 to co-found the Counseling Co-op in the Oak Lawn area of Dallas.

E. Tyronne Howze, M.A., moved to San Francisco, where he is currently the Program Coordinator of Operation Recovery for Operation Concern, a nonresidential drug program for gay men. Operation Concern is a multiservice organization that provides, in addition to its drug-recovery programs, psychotherapy, HIV/AIDS services, and support services to differently abled and elderly lesbians and gay men.

Rodney Holcomb is currently a Client Services Manager for Dallas's AIDS/ARMS Network, an organization that provides case management and coordination of area services to HIV-infected individuals and their families. In addition to having his own caseload, he supervises four other case managers, each of whom assists forty to sixty HIV-infected clients.

Arlene N. Hess-Dick, M.Ed., is no longer directly involved with Oak Lawn Community Services but continues her private practice in Richardson, Texas, and facilitates workshops on subjects related to loss psychology and death and dying issues. As her new last name shows, she has (happily) remarried.

Rev. Ted Karpf left St. Thomas the Apostle Episcopal Church to accept a position with the Public Health Service as the country's first HIV/AIDS Program Specialist, a position that is now included in each PHS region. In 1991, he was honored by the Assistant Secretary of Health with a Special Recognition

Award for "leadership in helping the nation prevent and alleviate pain, suffering, and death associated with HIV/AIDS." In early 1992, Ted resumed the duties of an active priest in the Diocese of Washington, D.C., and works as Liaison Manager for the CDC's National AIDS Clearinghouse.

Lizabeth Stephens Shelby, R.N., after several years in Tyler, Texas, has returned to Dallas, where she is the Director of Total Quality Management for the Cedars Mental Health Center. She is happily raising her two-year-old (as of 1992) daughter.

Tara Rowe, R.N., became pregnant during the time she was writing her chapter for this book and subsequently became less involved with both HIV-related volunteer work and her nursing career. Currently, she is a full-time mom.

Bill Edwards's lover, Art, died on May 6, 1987. Bill, who remains HIV-negative, lives alone but remains active in several organizations in and around Dallas that assist PWAs.

Gary Swisher has become Oak Lawn Community Service's Public Information Officer and Education Director. He was one of the founding members of the Texas AIDS Network, which he served as Chairman and then, until recently, as a Director. He is now the Chairman of the Texas HIV Health Care and Drug Fraud Task Force.

Ted Eidson moved from Dallas to Harlingen, Texas, in 1990 to accept the position of Executive Director of the Valley AIDS Council, the only AIDS service organization in the impoverished 4,300-square-mile southmost area of Texas, along the U.S./Mexico border. He has become a frequent speaker on issues dealing with HIV in Hispanic and rural communities, writes the "Fraud!" column for the *Texas AIDS Network News,* and is a member of the National Advisory Committee of The ARC (previously the Association of Retarded Citizens of the United States).

APPENDIX A

When a Friend Has AIDS

by Dixie Beckham, Luis Palacios,
Vincent Patti and Michael Shernoff

While serious illness is a fact of everyday life, AIDS has posed new challenges for everyone involved: not only individuals with AIDS, but also their friends and families. People who are in the prime of their lives have become ill, and their prospects for a long life have been severely affected. Their suffering and fear is shared by the people close to them.

When someone you know becomes ill, especially with a serious illness like AIDS, you may feel helpless or inadequate. If he or she has been a good friend you may say, "Just call if you need anything." Then out of fear or insecurity you may dread the call, if it comes. Here are some thoughts and suggestions that may help you to help someone who is very ill.

—Don't avoid her. Be there—it instills hope. Be the friend, the loved one you've always been, especially now when it is most important.

—Touch him. A simple squeeze of the hand or a hug can let him know that you still care. (Don't be afraid . . . you can not contract AIDS by simply touching.)

—Call before you plan to visit. She may not feel up to a visitor that day. Don't be afraid to call back and visit on another occasion. She needs you. She may be lonely and afraid.

—Weep with him when he weeps. Laugh when he laughs. Don't be afraid to share these intimate experiences. They can enrich you both.

—Call and say you're bringing her favorite dish. Be specific about what time you are coming. Bring the food in disposable containers, so she won't worry about washing dishes. Spend time sharing a meal.

—Take him for a walk or outing, but ask about and know his limitations.

—Offer to help answer any correspondence with which she may have difficulty dealing.

—Call and ask for a shopping list and make a "special delivery" to his home.

—Help him celebrate holidays—and life—by decorating the home or hospital room. Bring flowers or other special treasures. Include him in your holiday festivities.

—Help the lover, care-partner, spouse or roommate. Though she is the one who is sick, they may also be suffering. Care-partners may also need a small break from the illness from time to time. Offer to stay with the person who is sick in order to give the loved ones a break. Invite them out. Offer to accompany them places. They may need someone to talk with as well.

—Help care for the children. Offer to bring them to visit. Even if he's gay he may be a parent.

—Be creative. Bring books, periodicals, taped music, a poster for the wall, home baked cookies or delicacies to share with visitors. All of these become especially important now. Bring along another old friend who perhaps hasn't yet been to visit.

—Don't be reluctant to ask about the illness. She may need to talk about her condition. Find out by asking: "Do you feel like talking about it?"

—Don't feel that you both always have to talk. It's okay to sit together silently reading, listening to music, watching television . . . holding hands. Much can be expressed without words.

—Can you take him somewhere? He may need transportation to a treatment . . . to the store or bank . . . to the physician . . . or perhaps to a movie or community event.

—Help her feel good about her looks if possible. Tell her she looks good, but only if it is realistic to do so. If her appearance has changed, don't ignore it. Acknowledge the fact. But be gentle, and remember . . . never lie.

—Include him in decision making. He's been robbed of so many things and has lost control over many aspects of his life. Don't deny him a chance to make decisions, no matter how simple or silly they may seem to you.

—Tell her what you'd like to do for her, and if she agrees to it, keep any promises you make.

—Be prepared for him to get angry with you for "no obvious reason," although you've been there and done everything you could. Permit him this, and don't take it personally. Feel flattered that he is close enough to you to risk sharing his anger and frustration.

—Gossip with her if she indicates that she's tired of talking symptoms, doctors and treatments. If she seems interested, fill her in on family, clubs, organizations or mutual friends. Take your cues from her.

—What's in the news? Discuss current events with him. Help keep him from feeling that the world is passing him by.

—Offer to do household chores, perhaps taking out the laundry, washing dishes, watering plants, feeding and walking pets. This may be appreciated more than you realize. However, don't take away chores he can still do. He's already lost enough. Ask before doing anything.

—Send a card that says simply "I care!"

—If you are religious, ask if you could pray for her, or with her. Don't be hesitant to share your faith. Spirituality can be very important at times such as these.

—Don't lecture him or be angry if he seems to be handling the illness in a way that *you* think is inappropriate. He may not be where *you* expect or need him to be.

—Don't permit him or her to blame themselves for this illness. Remind them that lifestyles don't cause diseases, germs do. Help them through this one. It may be especially hard.

—If you two are going to engage in sex, be informed about the precautions which make sex safer for both of you. Heed them! Be imaginative . . . touch, stroke, massage. Sex need not always be genital to be fun.

—Remember that for gay men friends and lovers are also families. Demonstrate this by behaving like a loving family member if you are a friend, and by acknowledging the importance of these relationships if you are "blood" family or health care professionals.

—Do not confuse acceptance of the illness with defeat. This acceptance may free her and give her a sense of her own power.

—Don't allow him or the care-partner to become isolated. Let them know about the support groups and other concrete, practical services offered without charge by local AIDS service provider organizations.

—Talk about the future . . . tomorrow, next week, next year. Hope is important to her.

—Bring a positive attitude. It's catching.

Though these thoughts are meant primarily for people affected by AIDS, they are relevant to all who are seriously ill, because illness is part of the human condition. These suggestions have been adapted to the specialized needs of people with AIDS by the authors.

The authors work together at Chelsea Psychotherapy Associates, a group practice of New York State Licensed social workers located in Manhattan and founded in 1983. They are also volunteers at Gay Men's Health Crisis, the world's oldest and largest AIDS service provider organization.

Evidence of Lack of HTLV-III Transmission Among Families

by Kris Macdonald, M.D.

Nine studies have evaluated the transmission of Human T-Lymphotropic Type III (HTLV-III), also known as the AIDS virus, among family members of infected persons. Four of these studies have been published. For the other 5 studies summary data have been presented at scientific meetings or provided by the authors. Because of concern regarding the risk of HTLV-III transmission via casual contact, here is a summary of the 9 studies.

101 HTLV-III positive persons (index patients) in 8 of these studies were identified. The number of infected index persons included in one of the studies is not currently available from the authors; however, all were over 6 years old. In the 9 studies, at least 316 family contacts were evaluated for the presence of HTLV-III antibody to determine possible HTLV-III transmission in the household.

A total of twenty-one children less than 5 years of age were identified with HTLV-III infections. At least 71 family members of these 21 children were evaluated; 16 family members were less than or equal to 5 years old, 9 were 6 to 18 years old and 46 were adults. None of these contacts were HTLV-III antibody positive except for the adults or children who were also at high risk (i.e., adults who were intravenous drug abusers or sexual contact of HTLV-III antibody positive persons and children born to HTLV-III infected mothers). In one study, HTLV-III transmission was not demonstrated among child contacts of children infected with HTLV-III, even when intimate household activities, such as the sharing of toothbrushes and taking baths together, were included. Children under the age of 5 are probably the most likely of all infected persons to transmit HTLV-III through casual person-to-person contact because of their lack of control of secretions and poor personal hygiene.

To date, no AIDS cases have been identified among household contacts of the more than 13,500 cases of AIDS reported to the Centers for Disease Control. In addition, recent studies have demonstrated a very low risk of HTLV-III transmission from infected patients to health care workers (even workers who have had documented exposures to body fluids, such as needlesticks and mucosal exposures, from AIDS patients). All of these data support the conclusion that transmission from casual person-to-person contact is extremely rare, if it occurs at all.

In addition, a soon to be published study in a French boarding school for more than 100 boys with medical problems or handicaps has shown no spread of the AIDS virus in such a setting. The Pasteur Institute in Paris reported this finding in the group which includes some 50 boys with hemophilia, half of whom have evidence of AIDS infection and who sleep in the same dormitories, share meals and attend classes together. The children were between 3 and 16 years of age and have lived together for 1 to 3 years. None of the other 70 children have been infected with the AIDS virus even though the hepatitis B virus (HBV) was transmitted to some healthy classmates from hemophiliac students who are carriers of HBV. This latter finding suggests that an exchange of blood occurred between the students probably through scratches on their hands. The students thus had extremely close (household type) contact with one another but were still unable to transmit the AIDS virus.

Two cases reports suggest that HTLV-III/LAV infection may, on rare occasions, be transmitted during unprotected contact with blood or other potentially infectious body secretions or excretions in the absence of known parental or sexual exposure to these fluids. Adherence to published guidelines should prevent transmission through exposure to blood or body fluids.

Infection Precautions for Those Giving Direct Care to People with AIDS in the Home

Helen Schietinger, M.A., R.N.
Grace Lusby, M.S., R.N.
with input from UCSF AIDS Workers
and Bay Area APIC AIDS Resource Group

People caring for persons with AIDS in the home use standard precautions designed to prevent blood and other body secretions from entering the body through any body opening, including cuts or open areas on the skin. Handwashing before giving direct care protects the person who is susceptible to infection. Handwashing after direct care protects the caregiver.

Here are some specific precautions to use when giving direct care to someone with AIDS:

1. WASH YOUR HANDS. Hands do not need to be gloved for handling patient clothing and other articles that are not soiled. Hands do not need to be gloved to touch the patient's intact skin (for example, backrubs). Keep your hands away from mouth and face while working. Wash hands before eating.

2. Wear disposable gloves when handling any secretions or excretions, especially blood. Avoid direct skin contact with blood.

3. People who do not have AIDS can use the same bathroom as someone with AIDS. As in any living situation, good sanitary practices (not spilling excrement on toilet seats, etc. and cleaning the bathroom regularly) make it safe for everyone. Washing hands after use of the facilities is protective to others. Mopping of bathroom floor and cleaning of

other surfaces with standard household cleaning agents is sufficient for normal cleaning.

4. Dishes used by people with AIDS can be used by other people once they have been washed in hot soapy water. Allow to drain dry.

5. Kitchen floor and other kitchen surfaces can be cleaned using standard housecleaning agents. Sponges used to wash dishes and clean food preparation surfaces should not be used to clean other surfaces. Sponges and mops used to clean the floor should not be rinsed in food preparation sink.

6. Wash soiled linens and towels in a washing machine using the hot water cycle and detergent. Dry on high in dryer.

7. As you see, the surfaces and utensils used by a person with AIDS normally only require standard cleaning practices. Even used kitchen utensils are adequately cleaned when washed in hot soapy water, and the washing machine on the hot cycle will clean clothes and linens.

Surfaces (toilets, counters, floors) which have been *visibly* soiled with blood, fecal material or other body secretions, on the other hand, require disinfection. Household bleach is the best disinfectant because it is effective not only against AIDS but against organisms not killed by other household disinfectants (For example, use on the tub or shower floor as directed to control the fungus which causes Athlete's foot).

In order to use bleach safely, follow these instructions:

a. Wearing gloves and using paper towels, remove soil and disease causing organisms, washing with hot water and the appropriate household cleaning agent (detergent, scouring powder, etc.)

b. Following cleaning, rinse surface to remove all soap or other cleaning agent

    c. Apply a bleach solution to the surface *(¼ cup bleach to 1 gallon water).* This strength is sufficient to disinfect against AIDS and other organisms; stronger solution will cause fumes which are harmful to the respiratory tract

    d. Bleach should *never* be combined with other cleaning agents because the resulting fumes can be extremely harmful

8. When your clothing is likely to be in contact with secretions/excretions wear a gown, lab coat, or smock.

9. Use plastic bags to dispose of soiled tissues, dressings, bandages, and soiled gloves. Close and secure the bag tightly when discarding. Needles and other sharp items should be placed in puncture-resistant containers before discarding. Dispose of the bag in the garbage, as you would other solid waste.

10. Bedpans and urinals should be handled in a sanitary manner. Excrement need not be treated before being flushed down toilet.

11. Diarrhea and vomitus: Using gloves, clean up patient and linens immediately. Put soiled linens in plastic bag until ready to launder. Clean and disinfect surfaces as above, placing disposable items in a plastic bag as above.

12. Pregnant women are sometimes advised to avoid direct physical contact with people with AIDS because patients may be shedding CMV virus in body secretions. (CMV may cause birth defects.) However, if someone caring for a person with AIDS becomes pregnant, having used the listed precautions will have provided more protection against CMV than we ordinarily have in our daily contact with people, some of whom may be asymptomatic excreters.

13. AIDS is not transmitted through the air. However, a person with AIDS who has an active and persistent cough may

harbor other organisms which could be spread by the air-borne route. The main concern to healthy caregivers is the possibility of the cough being caused by TB. The other respiratory diseases that people with AIDS get are usually only of importance to people who are immunosuppressed. Should a cough develop, ask patient to cough or sneeze into a tissue or handkerchief, not directly into the air.

14. At the end of physical care, WASH YOUR HANDS. Use lotion on clean hands. (Clean hands will not contaminate lotion bottle.) Lotion is important to replace the natural oils removed by handwashing. Dry, chapped hands leads to open areas through which disease-causing organisms may enter. In addition, those areas may develop mild infections which could then be transmitted to the patient.

Revised 9/86

APPENDIX B

Getting Your Affairs in Order

by Michael Helquist

■ WHAT IS AIDS? ■

Presented here is our current understanding of AIDS, reflecting the best medical information available.

AIDS stands for **Acquired Immune Deficiency Syndrome**.
Acquired: To indicate that it is not an inherited or genetic condition, but is associated with the environment.
Immune: The immune system is the body's natural ability to protect against infection and disease.
Deficiency: Incomplete or lacking.
Syndrome: Characteristic combination of signs and symptoms.

Thus AIDS is an impairment of the body's ability to fight disease, leaving an individual susceptible to illnesses that the healthy immune system could protect against.

People with AIDS are susceptible to diseases known as "opportunistic conditions" because the individual cannot fight off some disease-causing organisms and certain tumors.

■ WHAT CAUSES AIDS? ■

Several theories are being investigated and many researchers believe that an infectious agent, probably a virus, is causing a breakdown of the immune system. It is further believed that this virus is carried in the blood or other body fluids (such as semen) and may be transmitted through intimate sexual contact, by sharing I.V. needles, or possibly by blood products. AIDS IS NOT TRANSMITTED BY CASUAL SOCIAL CONTACT.

Medical treatment of AIDS varies with the diseases involved. There has been some success in treating the diseases themselves and the arrest of further immune collapse. As yet, there is no effective treatment to rebuild the immune system and reverse the immune deficiency.

Getting your affairs in order relates to living well, to being as prepared as possible for unexpected events, and to protecting your interests as well as those of the special people in your life.

Have you successfully completed a contingency plan for your own benefit and that of your survivors? Can you afford to delay any longer such important planning?

This brochure has been developed by the San Francisco AIDS Foundation to assist you in your planning. Enclosed is also a worksheet form for your use in gathering your important personal information.

THE PRIMARY PURPOSE FOR GETTING YOUR AFFAIRS IN ORDER IS TO PROVIDE PEACE OF MIND FOR YOURSELF AND TO ENSURE MINIMAL DIFFICULTIES FOR THE SIGNIFICANT PEOPLE IN YOUR LIFE.

Your peace of mind can be enhanced by knowing that unforeseen developments will not totally disrupt your life.

Consider:

If you were in a serious but not fatal accident, would your lover, roommate, or friend know whom to contact?

If necessary, could you find out quickly what coverage your health insurance provides?

If your wallet or purse were lost or stolen, would you have a record of your credit cards, licenses, other important information?

If you are confronted with a life-threatening illness, do you need to worry as well about what financial difficulties you may be leaving to your lover, parents, and family?

Your preparations can make it easier for the significant people in your life to help you in emergencies and can ease their burdens should they become your survivors.

Consider:

How much difficulty would there be for your lover, roommate, or friends if you were temporarily hospitalized and were unable to maintain your daily routine?

If you were to die, would your survivors have to spend months trying to find your important, personal papers, trying to settle your estate? Would they have to close out your home without knowing your intentions?

Other Considerations:

Who do you want to have copies of this information?

Have you listed all your special possessions in your will? You may want to take a notebook and walk around your home listing your most cherished possessions. Next to each item list the name of the person to whom you would have liked to give it, had you died yesterday.

Do you want to add another person's name to your bank accounts, safe deposit box?

Do you want to change the beneficiary on any of your insurance policies?

If you have a collection of personal correspondence, a journal, or private papers, whom do you want to have these? Do you want these papers preserved or archived?

In case of emergency or death, do you want certain out-of-town friends or relatives to be notified? Who?

Do you want another person to have a set of keys to your home or car?

It could be very helpful to include with these forms and your will a copy of the current employee handbook listing the benefits for which you are eligible.

You may have already completed a contingency plan to protect yourself and others. Perhaps you can encourage someone you care about to do the same. For someone with a life-threatening illness, contingency planning may seem ominous. While acknowledging these feelings, you can provide support and assistance with gathering information.

■ GETTING YOUR AFFAIRS IN ORDER A WORKSHEET ■

Your Name: _____

Address: _____

Telephone: _____

Social Security Number: _____

Birthdate: _____

■ IN CASE OF EMERGENCY CONTACT ■

Name: _____

Address: _____

Telephone: (h) _____ (w) _____

Nearest Relative:

Name: _____

Telephone: (h) _____ (w) _____

■ RESOURCE CONTACTS ■

Employer: _____

Telephone: _____

Doctor(s): _____

Telephone: _____

Attorney: _____

Telephone: _____

Accountant/Bookkeeper: _____

Telephone: _____

■ FINANCIAL ■

Checking account

Bank: _____

Branch: _____

Acct. #: _____

Savings account

Bank: _____

Branch: _____

Acct. #: _____

Credit union

Branch: _____

Account #: _____

Other

Certificates: _____

Stocks, bonds: _____

Retirement Accts.: _____

_____

_____

Real Estate: _____

How title is held: _____

Loans to others: _____

■ DOCUMENTS ■

Will

Location: _____

Date: _____

Rental/Lease Agreement

Location: _____

Deposits to be returned: _____

Tax Records

Location: _____

■ INSURANCE COVERAGE ■

Health Insurance

Name of Company: _____

Address: _____

Telephone: _____

Agent/contact: _____

Life Insurance

Name of Company: _____

Address: _____

Telephone: _____

Agent/contact: _____

Disability Insurance

Name of Company: _____

Address: _____

Real Estate Documents

Location: _____

Safe Deposit Box

Location: _____

Location of key: _____

Who has access to box: _____

Vehicle Registration: # _____

Location of forms: _____

Vehicle License: # _____

Other Documents: _____

Telephone: _____ Car loan: _____

Agent/contact: _____

Auto/Home/other insurance Personal: _____

Name of Company: _____

Address: _____ Other: _____

Telephone: _____

Agent/contact: _____

Name of Company: _____

Address: _____ ■ **CREDIT ACCOUNTS/CARDS** ■

Telephone: _____ VISA/Mastercharge/other:

Agent/contact: _____

_____ # _____

_____ # _____

Deficits

Loans: _____ # _____

Mortgage: _____

_____ # _____

Dept. stores/gas cards:

Item   Person's Name

\# _____ _____ _____

\# _____ _____ _____

\# _____ _____ _____

\# _____ _____ _____

\# _____ _____ _____

\# _____ _____ _____

\# _____ _____ _____

■ MISCELLANEOUS ■

Possessions to be listed in your will that you would like
special individuals to receive:

Item   Person's Name   Who has copies of this form:

_____ _____ _____

_____ _____ _____

_____ _____ _____

                                     _____

Rights of People with AIDS

People with AIDS Have the Right:

1. To quality medical treatment and quality social service provision without discrimination of any form, including sexual orientation, diagnosis, economic status, or age.

2. To full explanations of all medical procedures and risks, to choose or refuse their treatment modalities, to refuse to participate in research without jeopardizing their treatment, and to make informed decisions about their lives.

3. To privacy, to confidentiality of medical records, to human respect, and to choose who their significant others are.

4. To as full and satisfying sexual and emotional lives as anyone else.

5. To live and die in dignity.

Medical Consent Form
(Sample)

I, _____ , being fully competent and having the legal capacity to consent to my own medical care, authorize _____ to consent to any x-ray examination, anesthetic, medical or surgical diagnosis or treatment, and medical care in the event that I become physically or mentally unable to give such consent.

Be it further known that is my_____ (fill in relationship, e.g., companion-in-life, business partner, close friend, etc.), and is to be afforded all of the privileges given to closest relatives and kin, including but not limited to scheduled visitation hours, 24-hour visitation in intensive care and elsewhere where allowed, access to information about my condition by consultation with hospital staff or by telephone, rooming-in, and full disclosure of all aspects of my condition.

Dated at _____ , _____ , 19__ .

_____
Signature

State of _____

County of _____

On this day personally appeared before me _____ , known to me to be the individual described herein and who executed the within and foregoing instrument, and acknowledged that s/he signed the same as a free and voluntary act and deed for the uses and purposes therein mentioned.

GIVEN under my hand and official seal this ____ day of ____ ,
19__ .

_____
Notary Public in and for the
State of _____
residing at _____

*This is a sample form. Check with local legal counsel for wording appro-
priate for your area.*

Solemn Statement Regarding Death
(Sample Living Will/Directive to Physician)

To my family, physician, lawyer, and other concerned persons:

If the time comes when I can no longer take part in the decisions for my own future, let this statement stand as a testament of my wishes:

If there is no reasonable expectation of my recovery from physical or mental disability, I request to be allowed to die naturally and not be kept alive by artificial means or heroic measures. Death is as much a reality as birth, growth, maturity, and old age. It is the one certainty. I do not fear death as much as I fear the indignity of deterioration, dependence, and hopeless pain. I ask that drugs for the relief of pain be mercifully administered to me for terminal suffering, even if they hasten the moment of death.

This request is made while I am in good health and spirits. Although this document is not legally binding, you who care for me will, I hope, feel morally bound to follow its mandates. I recognize it places a heavy burden of responsibility upon you, and it is with the intention of sharing that responsibility and of mitigating any feelings of guilt that this statement is made.

Dated: _____ Signed: _____

On _____ (date), at _____ (city and state), _____ (name) in our presence read the foregoing statement, declared it to express his/her wishes and subscribed his/her name to it, and requested each of us to attest to these facts as witnesses, whereupon in each other's presence, we sign this instrument.

Signatures: Addresses:

_____   _____

                                                _____

_____   _____

                                                _____

Subscribed and sworn before me this ____ day of ____ , 19__ .
Notary Public in and for the State of _____ ,
residing in _____ .

_____
Signature of Notary

This is a sample form. Exact forms for each state are available through The Society for the Right to Die (See Appendix E) or your attorney.

APPENDIX C

Generic List of Local and National Groups

There are a number of resources available to you within your own community. The list that follows is designed to help you locate the agencies and groups in your area by advising you of the *types* of those that have been helpful in the rest of the country. If a local agency is unable to offer assistance, they should be able to refer you to a group that can.

American Cancer Society
American Red Cross
Bookstores: general, metaphysical, gay, medical, etc.
Charity Hospital
Churches and Religious Organizations
Community Chest/Community Council
County/State Health Department
County/State Welfare Department
Crisis Intervention/Suicide Prevention Hotline
Gay Information Hotline
Gay Support Groups
Hemophilia Society
Libraries: public, colleges, medical schools
MHMR (Mental Health/Mental Retardation Assn.)
Narcotics Anonymous
Social Security Administration
U. S. Senators' and Representatives' Offices
United Fund/United Way
Veterans Administration
Visiting Nurse Association

National Telephone Hotlines

AIDS Clinical Trials Information Service, Public Health Service; (800) TRIALS-A = (800) 874-2572, or for the deaf, (800) 243-7012 (TTY), and international (301) 217-0023.

AIDS Hotline, Public Health Service, U. S. Department of Health and Human Services; (800) 342–AIDS.

AIDS Information Hotline, National Gay Task Force; (800) 221–7044 or (212) 807–6016.

National Sexually Transmitted Disease Hotline, American Social Health Association; (800) 227–8922.

Other Sources of Information and Referrals

National AIDS Network, 1012 14th. St., N.W., Washington, D.C. 20005; (202) 347–0390 (referrals to local groups).

National Association for People with AIDS, P.O. Box 65472, Washington, D.C. 20035; (202) 483–7979 (lobbying group for PWAs and referrals to local chapters).

Project Inform; (800) 822–7422 (medical and experimental treatment information derived from PWAs throughout the country).

Society for the Right to Die, 250 W. 57th St., New York, NY 10017; (212) 246–6973 (living Wills/directives for physicians for each state, legal information on right-to-die issues).

Spellman Center; (212) 307–0735 (general information for NYC area, considered by some more informative than CDC).

APPENDIX D

APPENDIX D

Reading List

Note: This reading list was compiled in 1988 for the first edition. The number of excellent books that have been printed since then on AIDS, death and dying, metaphysics and spirituality, stress, etc., is staggering. Check with your local bookstore. The ones listed here are the classics and are still in print.

Alexander, Thea. *Twenty-one Fifty, A.D.* New York: Warner Books, 1976 $3.95, paperback.   —— fiction

Bach, Richard. *Illusions: The Adventures of a Reluctant Messiah.* New York: Dell, 1977. $3.50, paperback.   —— fiction

Barnhart, Edward R. *Physician's Desk Reference.* Oradell, NJ: Medical Economics Books, annually. $29.95, hardcover.   —— drug encyclopedia

Benson, Herbert, and Klipper, Marian Z. *The Relaxation Response.* New York: Avon, 1976. $3.95, paperback   —— stress

Black, David. *The Plague Years: A Chronicle of AIDS, the Epidemic of Our Times.* New York: Simon & Schuster, 1985. $16.95, hardcover.   —— history

Boyd, Malcom. *Gay Priest: An Inner Journey.* New York: St. Martin's Press, 1986. $14.95, hardcover.   —— psychology

Carnes, Patrick, Ph.D. *Out of the Shadows: Understanding Sexual Addiction.* Minneapolis: CompCare Publications, 1983. $8.95, paperback.   —— sexual addiction

A Course in Miracles: Combined Volume. Tiburon, CA: Foundation for Inner Peace, 1985. $25.00, paperback. (1188 pages) — metaphysical workbook

Cousins, Norman. *Anatomy of an Illness as Perceived by the Patient.* New York: Bantam Books, 1981. $5.95, paperback. — self-healing

―――. *The Healing Heart: Antidotes to Panic and Helplessness.* New York: Avon Books, 1984. $3.95, paperback. — self-healing

Dalton, Harlan L., Burris, Scott, and the Yale AIDS Law Project, eds. *AIDS and the Law, A Guide for the Public.* New Haven and London: Yale University Press, 1987. $8.95, paperback. — law

Dass, Ram and Gorman, Paul. *How Can I Help? Stories and Reflections on Service.* New York: Alfred A. Knopf, 1987. $6.95, paperback. — caregiving

Davis, Chris. *Valley of the Shadow.* New York: St. Martin's Press, 1988. $13.95, hardcover. — AIDS fiction

Delaney, Martin, Goldblum, Peter, and Breuer, Joe. *Strategies for Survival.* New York: St. Martin's Press, 1987. $10.95, paperback. — workbook

Fletcher, David, M.D., M.P.H. "Positive AIDS Antibody Tests: What Do They Mean?" in *Medical Self-Care* Magazine, July–August, 1986, pp. 47–48. — medical

Gawain, Shakti. *Creative Visualization.* Mill Valley, CA.: Whatever Publishing, 1978. $7.95 paperback. New York: Bantam, 1978. $3.95, paperback. — visualization, alt. healing

―――. *The Creative Visualization Workbook.* Mill Valley, CA.: Whatever Publishing, 1982. $9.95, paperback.

visualization workbook

―――. *Living in the Light.* Mill Valley, CA.: Whatever Publishing, 1986. $8.95, paperback.

metaphysics

Gong, Victor. *Understanding AIDS: A Comprehensive Guide.* New Brunswick, NJ: Rutgers University Press, 1985. $10.95, paperback.

general

Gronewold, Sue. *Beautiful Merchandise: Prostitution in China: 1860–1936.* New York: Harrington Park Press, 1985. $7.95, paperback.

prostitution

Haas, Dr. Robert. *Eat to Win: The Sports Nutrition Bible.* New York: New American Library, 1985. $4.50, paperback.

nutrition

Hastings, Diana. *A Complete Guide to Home Nursing.* Woodbury, NY: Barron's Educational Series, Inc., 1986. $14.95, hardcover.

nursing

Hay, Louise. *Heal Your Body.* Santa Monica, CA: Hay House, 1984. $3.00, paperback.

alt. healing

―――. *You Can Heal Your Life.* Santa Monica, CA: Hay House, 1984. $10.95, paperback.

alt. healing

Humphry, Derek. *Let Me Die Before I Wake.* Los Angeles: Hemlock-Grove, 1986. $10.00, paperback.

euthanasia

Institute of Advanced Study of Human Sexuality. *Safe Sex in the Age of AIDS: Guidelines for Reducing the Risk of Contracting AIDS During Sexual Contact for Men and Women.* Secaucus, NJ: Citadel Press, 1986. $3.95, paperback.

safer sex

Institute of Medicine, National Academy of general
Sciences. *Mobilizing Against AIDS: The Unfinished Story of a Virus.* Cambridge, Mass.:
Harvard University Press, 1986. $7.95,
paperback.

Jampolsky, Gerrald G. *Love Is Letting Go of Fear.* spirituality
New York: Bantam Books, 1982. $3.50
paperback. Berkeley, CA: Celestial Arts,
1979. $5.95, paperback.

————, et al. *Goodby to Guilt: Releasing Fear* spirituality
Through Forgiveness. New York: Bantam,
1985. $8.95, paperback.

Keys, Ken, Jr. *Handbook to Higher Consciousness* metaphysics
(7th. ed.). Coos Bay, OR: Living Love, workbook
1985. $3.95, paperback.

Koop, C. Everett, M.D., Sc.D. *Surgeon Gen-* general
eral's Report on Acquired Immune Deficiency
Syndrome. Washington, D.C.: U. S. Department of Health and Human Services, un-
dated 1987. Free. Write: AIDS, Box
14252, Washington, D.C. 20044 or call
(202) 245–6867.

Kravette, Steve. *Complete Relaxation.* Glouces- stress
ter, MA: Para Research, Inc., 1979. $10.95,
paperback.

Kübler-Ross, Elisabeth. *Death: The Final Stage* death and
of Growth. New York: Simon & Schuster, dying
1986. $6.95, paperback.

————. *On Death and Dying.* New York: Mac- death and
millan/Collier Books, 1970. $4.95, paper- dying
back.

Kushner, Harold S. *When Bad Things Happen to Good People.* New York: Avon Books, 1983. $5.95, paperback.

philosophy

Lessing, Doris. *The Memories of a Survivor.* New York: Alfred A. Knopf, 1974. Out of print.

fiction

———. *Shikasta: Canopus in Argos-Archives.* New York: Alfred A. Knopf, 1979. $13.95, hardcover.

fiction

Levine, Stephen. *A Gradual Awakening.* New York: Anchor-Doubleday, 1979. $5.95, paperback.

death and dying

———. *Meetings at the Edge: Conversations with the Grieving and the Dying, the Healing and the Healed.* New York: Anchor-Doubleday, 1984. $7.95, paperback.

death and dying

———. *Who Dies? An Investigation of Conscious Living and Conscious Dying.* New York: Anchor-Doubleday, 1982. $9.95, paperback.

death and dying

McCarroll, Tolbert. *Morning-Glory Babies.* New York: St. Martin's Press, 1988. $14.95, hardcover.

children and AIDS

Mandel, Bea, and Mandel, Byron. *Play Safe: How to Avoid Getting Sexually Transmitted Diseases.* Foster City, CA: Center for Health Information. $4.95, paperback.

safer sex

Moffatt, BettyClare. *When Someone You Love Has AIDS: A Book of Hope for Family and Friends.* Santa Monica, CA: IBS Press, 1986. $9.95, paperback. (Also available through Hay House.)

alt. healing

——, et al., eds. *AIDS: A Self-Care Manual.* general and
The AIDS Project of Los Angeles. Santa   for PWA
Monica, CA: IBS Press, 1987. $12.95,
paperback.

Monette, Paul. *Love Alone: Eighteen Elegies for*   poetry
Rog. New York: St. Martin's Press, 1988.
$13.95, hardcover.

Moody, Raymond A. *Life After Life.* New   near-death
York: Bantam, 1981. $3.95, paperback.   experiences

Morgan, Ernest. *Dealing Creatively with Death:*   burial
A Manual of Death Education and Sim-
ple Burial (10th. ed.). Brunsville, NC:
Cleo Press, 1984. $6.50, paperback.
(Available free through some funeral
homes.)

Nickell, Molli, ed. *AIDS: Spirits Share Under-*   metaphysics
standing and Comfort from the "Other" Side.
Los Angeles: Spirit Speaks, 1986. $9.95,
paperback.

Peck, M. Scott. *The Road Less Traveled.* New   spirituality
York: Simon & Schuster, 1980. $9.95,   and risking
paperback.

Preston, John, ed. *Hot Living: Erotic Stories about*   fiction,
Safer Sex. Boston: Alyson Pub., 1985.   safe sex
$7.95, paperback.   (gay)

—— and Swann, Glen. *Safe Sex: The Ultimate*   safe sex
Erotic Guide. New York and Scarborough,   (gay)
Ont.: New American Library, 1987. $8.95,
paperback.

Ring, Kenneth. *Heading Toward Omega.* New   near-death
York: William Morrow/Quill, 1985.   experiences
$6.95, paperback.

Roberts, Jane. *The Education of Oversoul Seven.*   fiction
Englewood Cliffs, NJ: Prentice-Hall, 1984.
$6.95, paperback.

————. *The Further Education of Oversoul Seven.*   fiction
Englewood Cliffs, NJ: Prentice-Hall, 1984.
$6.95, paperback.

————. *Oversoul Seven and the Museum of Time.*   fiction
Englewood Cliffs, NJ: Prentice-Hall, 1984.
$6.95, paperback.

Ryan, Regina, and Travis, John. *Wellness Work-*   stress, death
book: A Guide to Attaining High Level Wellness.   and dying
Berkeley, CA: Ten Speed Press, 1981.
$9.95, paperback.

Schaefer, Walt. *Stress, Distress and Growth.*   stress
Davis, CA: International Dialogue Press,
1978. $9.75, paperback.

Shilts, Randy. *And the Band Played On: Politics,*   history
People and the AIDS Epidemic. New York: St.
Martin's Press, 1987. $24.95, hard-
cover.

Segal, Jeanne. *A Personal Program to Speed*   alt. healing
Healing and Enhance Wellness. Van Nuys,
CA: Newcastle Pub. Co., 1983. Out of
print.

Selye, Hans. *Stress Without Distress.* New York: stress
New American Library, 1975. $3.50,
paperback.

Serinus, Jason, ed. *Psychoimmunity and the Heal-*   alt. healing
*ing Process: A Holistic Approach to Immunity
and AIDS.* Berkeley, CA: Celestial Arts,
1986. $9.95, paperback.

Shaffer, Martin. *Life After Stress*. Chicago: Con-   stress
temporary Books, Inc., 1978. $9.95, paper-
back.

Shelp, Earl E., Sunderland, Ronald H., and Man-   pastoral care
sell, Peter W. A., M.D. *AIDS: Personal
Stories in Pastoral Perspective*. New York,
The Pilgrim Press, 1986. $7.95, paper-
back.

Simonton, Carl, et al. *Getting Well Again*. New   alt. healing
York: Bantam, 1980. $4.50, paperback.

Simonton, Stephanie M., and Shook, Robert L.   alt. healing
*The Healing Family: The Simonton Approach to
Families Facing Illness*. New York: Bantam,
1985. $3.95, paperback.

Slaff, James I., and Brubaker, John K. *The   general
AIDS Epidemic: How You Can Protect Your-
self and Your Family—Why You Must*. New
York: Warner Books, 1985. $4.95, paper-
back.

Stone, Judith. "AIDS Volunteers," in *Glamour*   volunteer
Magazine. March, 1987, pp. 288 ff.   services

Warren, J. Mark. "Out of the Closet—The   general
Myths and Realities of AIDS," in *Police
Journal* Magazine, February, 1987, pp.
10–12.

Westburg, Granger E. *Good Grief*. New York: death and
Fortress Press, 1962. $1.95, paperback.   dying

Williams, Margery. *The Velveteen Rabbit, or How   fiction,
Toys Become Real*. Illustrations, William   spirituality
Nicholson. New York: Doubleday, 1922.
$7.95, hardback.

Cassettes

Adair, Margo. "For People With AIDS." San Francisco: Tools for Change. 2 cassettes, 4 meditations: $14.15
"Envisioning a Healthy Immune System"
"Healing and Treatment of Choice"
"Respite: Enlightening the Heart and Relieving Pain"
"Wise Self: Courage to Keep Up the Fight and/or Let Go"

Allen, Marcus. "Stress Reduction and Creative Meditations." Mill Valley, CA: Whatever Publishing. $10.95

"A Course in Miracles." Tiburon, CA: Foundation for Inner Peace. Set of 42 tapes: $140.00

Fisher, Sally. "AIDS: Anger Incorrectly Directed at the Self." Los Angeles: Northern Lights Alternatives. $10.95.

————. "Body Talk." Los Angeles: Northern Lights Alternatives. $10.95.

————. "Self Love." Los Angeles: Northern Lights Alternatives. $10.95.

Gawain, Shakti. "Creative Visualization." Mill Valley, CA: Whatever Publishing. $10.95.

Hay, Louise. "AIDS: A Positive Approach." Santa Monica, CA: Hay House. $10.00.

Miller, Emmett, M.D. "Awakening the Healer Within." Stanford, CA: Source Cassettes. 2 cassettes: $15.95.

————. "The Healing Journey." Stanford, CA: Source Cassettes. $10.95.

————. "Letting Go of Stress." Stanford, CA: Source Cassettes. $10.95.

Myss, Caroline M. "AIDS: Passageway to Transformation." The Master Series: Genesis. Walpole, NH: Stillpoint, Inc. $9.95.

Simonton, Carl. "Role of Belief in Cancer Therapy." Azle, TX: Simonton Cancer Center. 4-cassette set: $45.00.

Simonton, Steffani. "Relaxation and Mental Imagery as Applies to Cancer Therapy." Little Rock: Health Training and Research Center. $10.00.

Stupen, Dick. "Strong Immune System." Malibu, CA: Valley of the Sun Publishing. $9.98.

Sun, Patricia. "Well-Being Meditation." Berkeley, CA: Patricia Sun Tapes. $15.00.

Note: Rule of thumb for ordering tapes by mail is to add $1.50 for postage and handling (or call for exact amount). Out-of-state orders do not require sales tax; remember to include sales tax for in-state orders.

Addresses of Smaller Publishers and Cassette Distributors

Barron's Educational Services, Inc.
113 Crossing Park Drive
Woodbury, NY 11797

(800) 645–3476

(800) 257–5729 (in N.Y.)

Celestial Press
(subsidiary of Ten Speed Press)
P.O. Box 7123
Berkeley, CA 94707

(800) 841–2665
(415) 845–8414

Comp-Care (800) 328–3330
2415 Annapolis Ln. (612) 559–4800
Minneapolis, MN 55441

Contemporary Books, Inc. (312) 782–9181
180 N. Michigan Ave.
Chicago, IL 60601

Cleo Press
1901 Hannah Branch Road
Burnsville, NC 28714

Harrington Park Press (607) 722–7068
12 W. 32nd. Street
New York, NY 10001

Hay House (800) 654–5126
3029 Wilshire Blvd. #206 (213) 828–3666
Santa Monica, CA 90404

Health Training and Research (501) 663–5369
Center
P.O. Box 7237
Little Rock, AK 72217

Hemlock Society (213) 391-1871
P.O. Box 66218
Los Angeles, CA 90066

IBS Press (213) 450–6485
2339 28th. Street
Santa Monica, CA 20405

International Dialogue Press (916) 758–6500
P.O. Box 1257
Davis, CA 95617

Living Love Bookroom (800) 843–5743
790 Commercial Ave. (800) 331–4719 (in Cal.)
Coos Bay, OR 97420

Medical Economics Books (800) 223–0581
P.O. Box C–779, Pratt Sta. (201) 262–3030
Brooklyn, NY 11205

Northern Lights Alternatives (213) 669–5395
2303 Brownson Hill Drive
Los Angeles, CA 90068

Para Research, Inc. (617) 283–3438
85 Eastern Ave.
P.O. Box 61
Gloucester, MA 01930

Patricia Sun Tapes (415) 524–5795
P.O. Box 7065
Berkeley, CA 94707

The Pilgrim Press (212) 239–8700
132 West 31 St. Street
New York, NY 10001

Simonton Cancer Center (817) 444–4073
Tapes and Literature Dept.
P.O. Box 1055
Azle, TX 76020

Source Cassettes (415) 328–7171
Dept. M–176
P.O. Box W
Stanford, CA 94305

Spirit Speaks (213) 820–1260
P.O. Box 84304
Los Angeles, CA 90073

Stillpoint, Inc. (800) 874–4014
Box 640 (603) 756–3508
Meetinghouse Road
Walpole, NH 03608

Ten Speed Press
P.O. Box 7123
Berkeley, CA 94707

(800) 841–BOOK
(415) 845–8414

Tools for Change
Dept. P
P.O. Box 14141
San Francisco, CA 94114

Valley of the Sun Publishing
Box 38
Malibu, CA 90265

(818) 889–1575

Whatever Publishing
P.O. Box 137
Mill Valley, CA 94941

(415) 472–2100

Subscriptions

AIDS Treatment News
P.O. Box 411256
San Francisco, CA 94141
(415) 282–0110

Up-to-date information on experimental drug testing, protocol for admissions, info. on results, etc. Also, what is happening in the underground and where. ($25.00/ quarter)

Project Inform
25 Taylor St., Suite 618
San Francisco, CA 94102
(800) 822–7422

Newsletter and information packages, as well as hotline service with information similar to "AIDS Treatment News." (Minimum $10.00 contribution)

PWA Coalition *Newsline*
263-A West 19th. St. #125
New York, NY 10011
(212) 627-1810

Monthly tabloid magazine "published by and for" PWAs and PWARCs. News from everywhere: political, social, human interest, fiction, etc. Acts as the unofficial newsletter for NAPWA (Nat'l. Assn. of PWAs). Complete updated resource listings for NYC area. An excellent way to learn which PWAs are doing what: And they are! (Minimum $20.00 contribution)

Focus: A Guide to AIDS Research
The AIDS Health Project
University of California at San Francisco
Box 0884
San Francisco, CA 94143
(415) 476-6430

Monthly publication presenting AIDS research information for health-care and service providers in readable format. Best synopsis of traditional medical, psychological, and epidemiological reports. ($36.00/yr.)

Health Resource Directory
Healthworks Media Systems, Inc.
P. O. Box 3014
Bayonne, NJ 07002
(201) 858-3030

Resources for cancer patients; it focuses on immune system stimulation; lists books, cassettes, videos, etc. Good for KS patients and those looking for immune system-enhancement ideas. ($5.95)

Workshops

The AIDS Mastery
Northern Lights Alternatives
2303 Brownson Hill Drive
Los Angeles, CA 90068
(213) 669-5395

For persons with AIDS or ARC and those people working with them. Focuses on the ability to create change in one's life. 2½ days. $250.

Being Powerful in the Face of AIDS
Dr. Robert Eichberg
1116 N. Robertson Dr., Su. 801
Los Angeles, CA 90048
(213) 659-2307

Getting in touch with how you are affected by AIDS, and how to move from immobility into power. Workshop can be structured for any type of audience. 1 evening. Price varies.

The Experience Weekend
Dr. Robert Eichberg
1116 N. Robertson, Su.801
Los Angeles, CA 90048
(213) 659-2307

Primarily gay participants with a number of relatives of gays. Focuses on taking responsibility for one's life and actions. 2 days. $295.

The Louise Hay Workshop
Hay House
3029 Wilshire Blvd. #206
Santa Monica, CA 90404
(213) 828-3666

An experimental healing session for PWAs, PWARCS, Worried Well, caregivers, and concerned public. 2 days. $225.

Patricia Sun Workshops
P. O. Box 7065
Berkeley, CA 94707
(415) 524-5795

Wide repertoire of workshops, all dealing with spiritual consciousness and with healing, though not specifically with AIDS. Length and price vary.

Note: The workshops above are some of the more widely recognized groups working on a nationwide basis. Check in your locale for information on workshops facilitated by local people: These are often just as beneficial and less costly. Prices shown may vary city to city; and special arrangements may be available to PWAs or special-interest groups.

INDEX